Doctor Patient and the Law

Doctor Patient and the Law

Poornima Advani

1998
BOOKS FOR ALL
Delhi-110052

Distributed By:
D K Publishers Distributors P Ltd.
1, Ansari Road, Darya Ganj,
New Delhi-110002
Phones: 3261465,3278368
Fax : 3264368
E-Mail: dkpd@del3.vsnl.net.in
Visit us at: www.dkpdindia.com

ISBN 81-7386-213-3

First Published 1998

Published By:
Books For All
B-2, Vardhaman Palace,
Nimri Commercial Centre,
Ashok Vihar Phase-IV,
Delhi-110052
Phone: 7401672
E-Mail: lpp@nde.vsnl.net.in
Visit us at: www.dkpdindia.com

Printed At:
D K Fine Art Press P Ltd.
Delhi-110052

PRINTED IN INDIA

The Ever Lasting

Ethical

Doctor - Patient Relation

Contents

Foreword

Dr. Poornima Advani has done it again!

That 'doing' consists in rendering, in many practical ways, relating the rule of law to what Pandit Nehru used to name as the 'rule of life.'

In all her published work so far, she has tried to demystify law and adjudication and raise concerns for the future of democratic law in India. Not content with the euphoria of the Golden Jubilee of Indian Independence, Dr. Advani biopsies the Indian futures.

From this point, this volume continues her quest. It is specifically addressed to the problems of law and medicine. And she brings very high credentials to this domain, being herself a singular practitioner of both in both the fields. Even as she summons the medical professions (I use the plural, given her insistence, and rightly so, that the practice of medicine is a 'joint enterprise' among the professionals and para-professionals) to its originary values, she interrogates, at times rather valiantly, the postures of contemporary Indian law, policy and administration in relation to ways of protecting the emergent consumer rights to human health, often grossly and at times subtly denied in the doctor-patient relationship.

Her canvas is, intimidating, vast. It addresses not just the local/

national law/medicine profiles, important as these are, but also the global developments in medical technology and practice which have not received sustained attention these deserve. Among these are global problems which visit Indian people rather severely, whether these be in the fields of artificial insemination practices, 'surrogate' motherhood, the AIDS or euthanasia. She makes, in each of these and related domains, visible the lack of critical discourse in India and alerts us to any mindless emulation of 'imported' discourses.

Dr. Advani is ruthlessly clear in her advocacy. That is the chief merit of her work. She is sceptical, both in terms of intention and impact, of subjecting the regimes of medical professions to the Consumer Protection Act. If at times she seems to valorize the medical professions and their 'nobility,' she also does not hesitate in insisting on patterns of more socially constructive regimes of self-regulation and where these might fail even more advanced forms of criminalisation of lapses in professional rectitude and integrity.

She displays considerable courage of conviction in essaying a critique of conversion of the learned medical professions into mere 'business' or 'occupations.' In doing so, she attempts a renaissance of cultures of medical practice in India and in particular draws attention of their reorientation towards an ethic of human rights.

The volume in your hands summons vigorous debate and contention on the nature of relationships between law and medicine, the rights and responsibilities of the medical establishment, the varieties of ways in which even the 'modern' law trembles into incoherence when confronted with runaway developments in science and technology and the ethical discourse at the heart of global industries capitalizing, as it were, human health and its problematic futures.

Dr. Advani is no Utopian theorist. She is 'pragmatic' in the very best sense of the term. She summons a national dialogue, informed by global controversies, on ways in which the Indian medical professions may move ahead in ways tinged, or even immersed, with social responsibility and concerns.

The fact that I differ from her in many aspects of her analysis and prescription (as may many of readers of this important work) is a tribute to her dialogical manner of presentation. And in this, I believe, lies the principal strength of her contribution to the contemporary bioethics debate.

I commend this significant endeavour to the two crucial professions - law and medicine - in order that these may reclaim their threatened statuses as 'learned' professions dedicated to human rights and amelioration of human suffering as ways of servicing the future of human rights in an obscenely globalising human future.

UPENDRA BAXI

PROFESSOR IN LAW AND DEVELOPMENT
WARWICK UNIVERSITY SCHOOL OF LAW
(Former Vice Chancellor
University of South Gujarat
and University of Delhi.)

Prologue

Medicine and law, although diverse fields, have much in common. Seemingly wide apart, they are yet intricately interwoven. Since times immemorial, these fields of learning have stood apart from the rest of the professions as segregated categories. In ancient times, placed on a high pedestal, these professions commanded great public awe and respect. Confidence and faith, by people at large, had been bestowed on them in abundance. In turn, both, the doctor and the lawyer, had shown deep concern for their patients and clients respectively, dedicating themselves to service of humanity and public wellbeing. So intimate was this interdependence, the interrelation of the doctor and his patient, the lawyer and his client, so ingrained was their interse faith that, with time, the two professions came to occupy a distinguished status, a stamp of nobility as if embossed on them. Within the framework of their duty towards their patients and clients and the superimposed stamp of nobility, the earning of livelihood had become and indeed was looked upon as merely a by-product of their activity. What really distinguished these two professions as a class apart was the fact that the predominant demand on them and the outcome of their duties was service to humanity, one set battered by sickness and disease, the other aggrieved by crime and injustice. Whether in reality everyone engaged in these two professions could make a living from the start or as to how many years it took them to attain the stage of a reasonable earning had never been an issue. It had also never been questioned whether every one of these professionals did treat service to humanity as paramount. No fixed norms of payment existed; it simply depended upon the goodwill and pocket of the beneficiary of their skill. The ingrained humanitarian firmament and the Hippocrates Oath,[1] would ring a bell at the right time to say: 'here comes your call of duty.' In fact, till very recently, the question whether any of them had come to be tainted by the polluted environment of society in general was itself a moot point.

Paradoxically speaking, the medical profession is the most self sacrificing occupation since, without fail, it has to work relentlessly for self immolation. Just pause and ponder. The doctor continuously, consistently and ceaselessly works and seeks to move towards the cure of the very disease which forms his bread and butter. Once the disease vanishes, so does his patient and incidentally his source of earning.

And what about the lawyer? In the days gone by, more specifically in the middle ages, barristers were known to wear their gowns with a pocket at the back where gracious clients would occasionally drop a few coins as a mark of gratitude. The fees were neither demanded nor settled prior to litigation. The lawyer's high sense of nobility would prevent him from peeping into his pocket. Only within the precincts of his home, away from the eyes of the world, would he feel the coins and get the satisfaction of having earned sufficient to provide meals for him and his. In the eighteenth century, the barrister could trace his proud lineage back to a stage when the pleader did not accept payment from clients; this is why the client's payment was an 'honorarium' instead of a 'fee.'[2] Nobility

---

[1]Hippocrates (about 460-377 BC) the most celebrated physician of antiquity, was born and practiced in the Island of Cos in Greece. He was the son of a physician and became so famous that (by common consent) he is regarded as the 'Father of Medicine.' The medical profession pay homage to Hippocrates by acknowledging the principles of the Hippocrates Oath to be worthy of emulation from the time they enter the portals of medicine: See Homi S. Mehta, *Medical Law and Ethics in India* 67 (1963) The Bombay Samachar Pvt Ltd.

[2]Lenard R Berlanstein, *The Barristers Of Toulouse in the Eighteenth Century (1740-1793)* 25 (1975) The John Hopkins University Press.

invariably locked his hands. Much later, the two fields, medicine and law, got stamped as professions. By their very nature, they affected human life or at least its quality. Specialised higher education, formal training, systematic and continuous advancement to keep pace with the developing technology became inevitable. Formation of professional associations, councils and institutions followed. For example, the General Council of the Bar was formed in 1895, as an elected body, with no disciplinary powers, but as a matter of practice, complaints were brought before it. The Indian Medical Council[3] and the Bar Council of India[4] were thus the outcome of pressing call for self-disciplinary codes. The Hippocrates Oath crowned the work of every doctor and the limitations of the '*sanad*' bound every lawyer, while their councils and associations disciplined them all. Thus it was that these two professions formed a class by themselves.

The difficulties and hurdles encountered by the two professions, medicine and law, have also been multifold. Take the medical stream. Intellectual supremacy is an essential ingredient even to enter the portals of the schools of learning. It requires high intellect coupled with economic sufficiency and hard labour to perform reasonably well, academically, to get admission into the

---

[3]The Indian Medical Council Act, 1956, was enacted to provide for the reconstitution of the Medical Council Of India and the maintenance of a Medical Register for India. Earlier, the Indian Medical Degrees Act, 1916, was meant to regulate the grant of title implying qualifications in western medical science and the assumption and use by unqualified persons of such titles.

[4]The Indian Bar Councils Act, 1726, was enacted in response to a demand by the legal profession for unification and autonomy of the Bar, and it did achieve a fair measure of both eliminating the two grades of practitioners, the vakils and the pleaders by merging them in the courts in which they were enrolled and in any other court in British India, subject to certain exceptions.

Prior to Advocates Act, 1961, there was no 'All - India' Bar Council. Each High Court had a Bar Council of its own : See Sanjiva Rao, The Advocates Act and The Legal Practitioners Act (1987) The Law Book Company (P) Ltd, Allahabad, India.

competitive medical stream. It then takes a number of years to qualify before one can even select a specific branch of specialisation and then perhaps a few more to crown it with super-specialisation which is indeed the demand of today. In practice, it takes an equal number of years and individual experience to acquire high calibre working skills and gain confidence of the patients/clients.

Ordinarily, a patient can never, truly and well, even know whether the professional expertise to which he has been subjected was called for, or whether it was imposed on him and could have been avoided. Even otherwise, the same surgeon can succeed or fail in similarly diagnosed cases, the same medicine may succeed with one and have no effect on another or yet harm a third. No two patients respond to the same line of treatment in the same manner and to the same degree. Mere will to recover, or the absence thereof, can brighten or mar the prognosis. In any case, no two patients or ailments can ever be identical. Still due to nature's inevitable vagaries and human being's pressing need of the moment, the patient simply surrenders his most precious possession, his body, and the spark of life within him, unconditionally to the doctor knowing that every disease, every treatment, carries its own risk. Life itself exists till it may. Any moment might be the last with or without medication. No doctor can guarantee or warranty life or even relief, notwithstanding his skill, knowledge, dedication and sincerity of purpose. The relationship between the doctor and the patient is one of goodwill and trust. Risk is an unavoidable ingredient of medical treatment and the doctor has to take it if at all he is to handle disease and injury and more so the serious or risky ones.

Likewise, in every litigation, there has to be a winner and a loser. Who wins, who loses, cannot be the yardstick of legal acumen or the measure of the lawyer's ability or the work put in by him. Best of the cases are lost and the worst ones many-a-time succeed. That is litigation and no lawyer can guarantee results, much less in today's times when even the portals of justice are besmirched.

However, whatever may have been the era, whatsoever the professional standing or the degree of acumen, the master key that has pervaded both sets of professionals is 'accountability' to the patient and/or the litigant. Paradoxically, on the one hand, stares out accountability and, on the other, the impossibility of guaranteeing success. One can visualise the predicament of a doctor, required to render service to a patient needing emergency care, without the back drop of any knowledge of the patient, his medical history, the allergies and above all his nature, as well as economic condition, knowing the risk to the patient's life and limb either ways, the expertise, knowledge and skill notwithstanding. Scaling the pros and cons between the need of the patient and the invariable risk involved a sensitive balance, often creating a tug-of-war situation, a fight between to-do or not-to-do. Indeed it is the most stress causing condition that the medical man has to face. Yet, millions must have been saved by the risks taken by these saviours of human lives.

Today, the doctor-patient relationship has come under serious stress which is becoming more and more precarious day by day. By the curbs, compulsions and coersions introduced within the relationship, the golden thread with which hangs the life of the sick and the wounded, is no longer handled by the doctor on the presumption of faith and trust. The traditional dominant role of the doctor has been hit by increasing number of ethical and legal challenges in the new era. When the entire nation is infected with materialism from top to bottom, when corruption has invaded the portals of parliament and sanctuaries of justice, when the poor have been made poorer by the umpteen scams involving hundreds of thousands of crores and the siphoning of uncountable monies abroad by violation of laws, when the foreign banks are bursting with ill-gotten wealth of the power-lords, is it possible that the doctors and the lawyers alone will stand out as shining examples of self-sacrificing citizens? It cannot but be expected that the fever of materialism would have affected the nobility of these professionals too, at least to some extent. Yet, overlooking the age old respect the professionals enjoyed, and their practical difficulties, the movement of consumerism and the enthusiasm of the activists as if engulfing them taking a toll of the goodwill of the masses.

The recent years have seen the medical man having to face a volley of complaints for medical mishaps. These inflictions, howsoever essential or called for, have surely but steadily tilted the scales from the established norms of a relationship of faith and trust between the doctor and the patient. The worst part of the infliction clamped on a doctor comes from a different quarter. The media reporting of even a single case of complaint against a doctor, real or imaginary, correct or concocted, flimsy or frivolous, completely destroys his reputation and, incidentally, his will to do something for the patient whatever be the consequences.

Today, every patient is looked upon with fear as a potential 'commercial consumer' client who may turn out to be a mere pawn in the rivalry of a neighbour, or a hard nut who must have his pound of flesh if he is not cured, or an aggrieved litigant if he happens to be victim of an accidental mishap in the flight for life waged by the doctor by a risky treatment procedure. Rightly or wrongly, the professional services of doctors have become subject to examination by those not conversant with medical sciences. The Supreme Court ruling[5] that the Consumer Protection Act, 1986 (CPA) does take within its fold the medical fraternity has created a rising wave amongst the masses to sue the doctors for negligence, without going into the doctor's dilemma under which he has had to take an instant and important decision. The age-old adage that the right to take a decision is merely the second side of the coin holding the right to make mistakes is no longer applied to the

[5]*Indian Medical Association v V P Shantha and others*, AIR 1996 SC 550.

medical profession. And it is not difficult to attribute mistakes in retrospect. This state of affairs has, unfortunately, given rise to a frenzy amongst doctors who are becoming more and more sceptical about taking any risks to save human lives even in emergencies and have taken to intensive and extensive investigations as a pre-condition for prescribing even common drugs.

The Supreme Court has, by this decision, painted the doctors with the same brush as the traders, the businessmen and the like, and embossed the patients with the stamp of consumers, without an analysis of where this movement is going to lead the citizenry to. Services to human life have been now placed on par with services for production of goods, notwithstanding the major difference that life and health problems cannot stand any guarantees. The 'services' rendered by 'traders' meaning doctors, to 'consumers' meaning patients, are expected to bear guarantee of 'workmanship' and production of results meaning 'life and cure.'

Yet the challenges to the medical faculty are getting more and more complex day by day. For example, medical scientists have been incessantly working towards improving the average life span of man and reducing death rate. A lot has been achieved but under the promise of prolonged life, many a disease has had to be blanketed as 'terminal.' With life becoming more and more complicated, life span enhancing rapidly, and uncontrolled population explosion infesting the country, the medical fraternity is unable to keep pace with the ever-increasing demand. With the enormous poverty-stricken masses as also the sick and elderly forced by circumstances to live an economically and physically dependent life, unattended and uncared for, the medical aid needs to be enhanced tremendously if at all some compassion is due to them. The enormity of the very issue is indeed mind-boggling.

As a natural corollary, questions have begun to be whispered whether such burdensome persons should at all be aided to live or should they be allowed to die peacefully? The corollary issues are no doubt complex and perplexing, yet crucial and critical, made more so by the intervention of CPA, supposedly a cheap, easy and quick remedy, in the already heavily painted scenario of odds and ends.

As if to keep pace with rapid strides in the fields of medicine and medical biotechnology, legalists and activists have created many more basic issues and dilemmas paving the path for an urgent multi-disciplinary dialogue involving social, ethical and religious issues in the backdrop of legal aids, existing or needing introduction.

Some issues involving mixed questions of law and medicine vis-a-vis ethics have already raised explosive debates and outrageous opinions. First and foremost is euthanasia, a word which can scarcely be mentioned without arousing deep compassions, convictions and passion. The debates on feasibility of legal permissiveness to take away a life have only aided to make the issue an eternal enigma. Then comes abortion. A subject of criminal prosecution in some countries, a matter of inevitable ethics in others and the emergency need in the case of HIV infected mothers putting the unborn in danger of AIDS, are topics which concern doctors the most, but they being the 'law-illiterates,' no doctor knows what the law permits and/or prohibits. When the mishap occurs, they knock at the doors of the 'medicine-illiterates' and then the attempt to know the law and the legal loopholes and place them in juxtaposition of medicine begins; confusion-cum-chaos ensues.

More thought provoking is the newly created market for human organs. Should the sale be permitted even to save other lives? Transplant having succeeded in enhancing life span, is it a blessing since it saves a life doomed to death or is it a curse since it has already given place to commercialisation and popularisation of an organ bazaar, bringing the ever vulnerable poor and needy under the axe? Is not the very thought of obtaining an organ from another living being, taking advantage of his vulnerability born of poverty, a basic violation of human rights?

The legal issues that technological revolution in medicine have created are endless. As this book goes into print, comes news of 'designer baby' techniques in America being condemned by British Medical Association,[6] surgeons having transplanted monkey's heads on to fresh bodies paving the way for a new era in human transplant technology[7] and cloning of human organs facilitating them to be grown custom-made in laboratories.[8] The ultrasound test designed for detection of genetic disorders is being increasingly employed for gender determination and selective abortion of the female foetus in keeping with the craze for a male child in some countries. However, enumerations apart, an urgent call to bridge the gap between social logic, legal reasoning and medical technology can no longer be ignored. Of great significance is the thought-filled introspection as to how each of the professions could utilise their specialised knowledge to address the increasing needs of humanity. Today, doctors, lawyers, scholars, theologians, parliamentarians, et al are often found groping on related problems, looking at them from different dimensions and coming to equally varied solutions, many a time in conflict with one another, adding more chaos and confusion to the already complex scenario.

Physicians of today, convoluted in their own mesh of technical proficiency, are now being affronted with situations never encountered before. The complex innovations of science are being misused and mismanaged only to complicate the matters further. The cobwebs are getting intertwined, professed proficiency overwhelmingly filling the already compound bandwagon, raising several questions which seemingly defy solutions. For example:

---

[6]The Times of India (New Delhi ed.) 22 August 1997.

[7]The Times of India (New Delhi ed.) 10 November 1997.

[8]The Hindu (New Delhi ed) 21 October 1997.

- should an aged and critically ill patient in a comatose stage or in excruciating pain be made to live indefinitely through expensive life-sustaining modalities which could instead be used for other patients with the hope of survival or should he be allowed to die a peaceful death?
- should a foetus be carried to term and allowed to be born alive when sonography has revealed severe genetic abnormalities?
- should treatment be withheld to infants with incurable serious physical defects with no chance of survival? What if the parents, too, demand it?
- who should be bestowed with powers to take decisions in an environment of clouded moral and ethical priorities? The medical professional, the legal professional, or, should these decisions lie with the patients on the basis of 'informed consent'? Or still, on their 'concerned' relatives?
- how far should the laws invade the ethico-medico standards of the medical profession, bearing in mind the desired confidentiality of the patient-doctor equation?
- where the patient is incapable of giving an informed consent, should legal intervention or advice to withhold life-prolonging treatment be regarded as a gratuitous trespass on the territory of the medical expert?

These and similar questions, having far reaching effects, need an urgent answer. In practical politics, every discovery in the field of medicine is seen to create fresh legal issues which require urgent debate and updating to settle the uncertainty. Inevitably, scientific advancements in medicine have given rise to complex and compulsive legal issues. The exigencies of a society demand that in the interest of humankind, law and medicine must correlate intricately and intimately.

For example, in the United Kingdom, Mr Patrick Steptoe

and Dr Robert Edwards extracted an ovum from Mrs Lesley Brown and fertilised it in a dish with her husband's semen. Incubated with great care with a special nutrient in their laboratory, it was then fertilised and the embryo was implanted in the uterus of Mrs Brown where it adhered and grew to full maturity resulting in the birth of Louise Brown on 24 July 1978.[9] The success of this experiment brought forth exciting prospects and opened up vistas of hope for the infertile couples. However, human ingenuity being what it is, experiments with the seeds of donors started multiplying, giving rise to a number of problematic issues like, who should be considered the father of the child - the man married to the lady who bore the child or the one who genetically was the giver of the offspring?

These developments gave rise to deep concern and sharp debates in Britain, as a result of which the government set up a Committee of Enquiry into Human Fertilisation and Embryology, in 1982, under the chairmanship of Lady Warnock and, two years later, the Committee presented its report to Parliament of United Kingdom highlighting about 65 recommendations.[10] Legalists had to step in to find some solution to these pragmatic 'medicine created complications' which had given rise to warring claimants of the newborns.

In an attempt to coordinate scientific developments and legal controls, the Committee pointed out that the advancement in medical technology in the field of human fertilisation had opened up new avenues for legal thinking. For example, invitro fertilisation had given rise to situations never before contemplated, with the result no legal provisions existed, necessitating fresh laws to cope

---

[9]Barbara Eck Menning, *A Guide for the Childless Couple* 83, 2nd ed (1977) Prentice Hall Press.

[10]Bernard Knight , *Legal Aspects of Medical Practice* 271, 5th ed (1992) Churchill Livingstone.

with these legal consequences flowing from the new techniques for alleviating infertility as also to deal with the research development in the field of embryology. However, while medical science has developed with startling rapidity to meet the demands of society, there is always resistance to the laws intervening specially in areas where there is absence of public consensus. Thus arises the need for systematic dynamic laws, as well as caution in their formulation, to keep pace with the rapid changes in development.

All said and done, suffering and injustice, the two fields requiring the services of medicine and law, continue to escalate creating stress and strain for humanity, claiming more and more lives. To actively aid in reducing, if not alleviating, the human misery ought to be our first and foremost concern. To match the ever-increasing demand for relief, the two professions are already under strain with medical science making swift advances and legal experts working round the clock to fit legislation into narrow grooves to meet every contingency. It is therefore necessary and in the interest of society to make a conscious attempt to understand and evaluate the difficulties of these professionals who also must continue to put in their very best, day in and day out, if at all they have to live upto their own conscience and satisfy the expectations of society from them. Obviously, the wide gap between the expectations of society on the one hand, and the limitations of the professionals on the other, affected to some extent by the materialism that has gripped the nation at all levels, has already resulted in enhanced litigation against the medical professional. The legal profession has, because of the very nature of their work field escaped so far except a few cases as, obviously, it is they who have to litigate on behalf of the aggrieved.

The immediate need of both the professions, law and medicine, as also the respective councils and associations, to glance with a disciplined and humanitarian look at the erring members of each faculty cannot, by any stretch of imagination, be underestimated. In today's world, self regulating instincts seem to have been blown off with the wind and discipline maintaining mechanisms have become rusty and ineffectual. It would be in the interest of the professions to do introspection, enter into their own soul searching chambers and adapt new strategies to re-enforce ethical standards.

Statistically speaking, being aware of the gross backlog of litigations before the courts in India,[11] speedy justice is a far cry. The staggering The Times of India (Bombay ed) 21 August 1995. pendency even in the consumer forums is fast becoming unmanageable, what with the addition of litigation involving medical matters without the CPA having provided any in-built knowledgeable paraphernelia for dealing with such cases.

The present strategy of the Consumer Redressal Forum to invite 'experts' from medical fields is laden with problems and pitfalls and is, to say the least, unsatisfactory and time-consuming. 'Experts' are known to be interested witnesses who must depose in favour of those who engage them. Their evidence is, quite often, untrustworthy. The system does not have the sanctity of legislation nor are there any rules and regulations for appointing experts. The whole procedure lacks credibility.

The interpretation of the provision that if the services are rendered free, then the giver of the services, medical or legal, cannot be hauled up under the Act, militates against social justice. For, free or paid, doctors deal with lives and not mere materials and they ought to be accountable to the patient and his near and dear ones for their negligence even though they may have treated a patient 'free'. There is no greater injustice in an equality professing country than to bar non-paying patients from the supposedly cheap,

---

[11]"About 25 million cases are pending in various courts in the country", according to Union Law Secretary Dr P.C.Rao: See, The Daily (Bombay ed) 8 November 1995.

easy and quick redressal avenues thus segregating the non-affording poor masses for non-redressal or in the alternative, knocking at the doors of civil and criminal courts. The whole idea stinks of injustice and cruelty to the poor needy of the country and leaves everyone with a big question mark - was the CPA really intended to cover medical services? This whole rigmarole and uncertainty could have been avoided if the legislation had, at every point of clearance, right from the stage of underlying objects to the drafting and passing of the statute, starting with definitions right upto the appointment of experts and representatives placed as members in the council, made this intention known and imposed the liability in clear terms.

However, facing the law as spelt by the courts, it is time to actively consider revamping the medical councils with more powers and introducing qualified experienced personnel in the councils formed under the CPA as a workable solution. The ideal, of course, would be the introduction of a seperate legislation applicable to professions and an Administrative Medical Tribunal like those for government servants and for motor accidents. There is absolutely no logical reason for clubbing professions with trade and commerce. An ideal body to try professionals should be multi-disciplinary, for example, a three or five member bench consisting of a retired member of the judiciary of the minimum rank of a high court judge, two doctor members and two social scientists would form a suitable panel. It would primarily be the duty of the judge to ensure fair proceedings. His legal acumen will be a sufficient safeguard for the legal fraternity. Technical and practical aspects could be dealt with by the other members. The faculty members would understand the issues raised, the evidence produced and the quality of witnesses, making the working of the consumer redressal forums easier and speedier.

The field correlating law and medicine is too vast to enable inclusion in this treatise wherein while dealing with both the fields, the intricacies have been omitted. In my association with all three sets who would be concerned with this subject matter, the medical man, the lawyer and the citizen-patient, I have had to often deal with the medical man caught in litigation, unaware of his rights and responsibilities under the laws and the basics of procedures, to convince him of a fair deal in the courts. I have had to elucidate the medical basics and terminologies to many a legal expert to enable him to appreciate the case of the medical man. And the citizen? Human physiology and legal principles are a tough matter to summarise usefully. Both are intricate sciences and in every single case, the slightest factual variation can have tremendous medical and legal implications. Still, in the general framework presented, attempt has been made to highlight some facets of the 'multi-dimensional' whole. Many questions remain. So it is where knowledge is concerned and so be it.

I do hope this treatise will be useful as a ready reckoner for the basics in medicine, law and general principles to the medical man, the lawyer and the citizen when confronted with the curse of litigation. In addition, it is intended to be an eye-opener for the consumer activist who, by their misguided activism, have done more harm to the masses than the good they had intended to do. For, all said and done, if the masses have to expect the best of services from the doctors, there is no point in "condemning as negligence that which is only a misadventure" and it is this caution projected by Lord Denning in *Roe v Minister* of Health[12] which has assumed significance in today's scenario. Or, else, not before it is too late, we would have these 'saviours' with their 'initiatives styled' and 'confidence shaken.'

[12] (1954) 2 QB 66, at 87.

Consumer Protection And The Medical Professional

Introduction

The escalating unfair trade practices in a customer-exploitable market, had led to a systematic deterioration in the quality of goods which had awakened the consumers to their serious handicaps in day to day life. Food poisoning, adulteration of life-saving drugs and similar calamitous conditions, at times fatal, were enjoined on the consumers with no easy mode of redress.

Advancement in the art of marketing management introduced by business houses had created a new set of organised commercial advertising agencies to aid the supplier with yet newer methodologies, raising the market persuasions and temptations to dizzy heights. The consumer, caught in the net spread out by the marketing experts, was an easy target of the enticing strategies. A study of the conditions, at that time, revealed a massive imbalance of equation between the user and the producer.

Prevailing laws were hardly effective in checking the gross violation of business ethics and non-observance of even the basics of commercial norms. *Caveat emptor,* meaning 'buyer beware,' had been voiced with no effect. A clarion call for reforms, audible and persistent, echoed from all four corners.

The voices had given rise to a strong consumer movement, which steadily demanded protection against the uncontrolled exploitation by the trader through unfair practices. Consumer activism was at its peak. The need to combat the situation could be contained no longer.

To protect the interest of an average consumer, to ensure for him qualitative performance by the traders, to clothe him with a right to compensation in case of defective goods or deficient services, had become essential. Soon tables would turn and the old yield place to new. The existing protocol of 'buyer beware' could not sustain itself any longer. Deftly and swiftly, the coin flipped to the other side.

In India, consumer awareness took a sudden leap and culminated in the enactment of the Consumer Protection Act, 1986[13] (CPA). Speedy trials, cheap modes of filing complaints, exemption from payment of court fees and informal procedures to facilitate the common man were the hallmark of this consumer oriented legislation.

The Consumer Protection Act, 1986

The preamble to the Consumer Protection Act, 1986, aimed basically at the protection of the consumers' interest.[14] To achieve the objective, a three tier quasi judicial machinery was sought to be set up at the central, state and district levels. Called Consumer Disputes Redressal Forums, these quasi-judicial bodies were empowered to grant specific relief and to award, wherever appropriate, compensation to consumers, while observing the

[13]This Act received the assent of the President of India on December 24, 1986, and came into force (with the exception of Chapter III) on April 15, 1987. Later, on July 1, 1987, Chapter III which deals with establishment of Consumer Disputes Redressal Agencies came into force. The Act has thereafter been amended in 1991 and still later in 1993.

[14]The Preamble, which sets out the main objectives of the Act states: "An Act to provide for better protection of the interests of consumers and for that purpose tc make provision for the establishment of consumer councils and other authoritie: for the settlement of consumers disputes and for matters connected therewith."

principles of natural justice in the discharge of their functions. In addition, the CPA also provided for penalties. However, the states, despite pressure exerted by consumer organisations, were rather slow, in setting up the redressal forums[15] and in fact, only the intervention of the Supreme Court of India[16] could accelerate the 'tardy and sluggish' States, into implementing the sanctioned measures. From the very inception of the forums, complaints relating to unfair trade practices started pouring in. The effect was immediate. The philosophy 'buyer beware' was replaced by 'seller beware.'

Not meant to be a full fledged commentary on the CPA, this chapter deals with only those provisions which favour or militate against the relevance of the Act to professionals and, in any case, need to be read as if applicable to them in view of the judicial interpretation thereof.

By and far, it can be asserted that, in India, till the disputes arose on the interpretation of CPA, the distinction between 'trade', 'commerce' and 'profession' had been maintained by governments as well as private bodies. The demarcation was clear-cut. No trader was a professional and vice versa, no professional could pass off as a trader.

For example, in the State of Maharashtra, an employment guarantee scheme was introduced about three decades ago. The proposal was to guarantee employment to the unemployed and collect the amount payable under the scheme by levying tax on those engaged in any earning venture. Since not only the trader and the professional were to be brought into the net but also those engaged in any other vocation, the Act was called The Maharashtra State Tax on Professions, Trades, Callings and Employment Act,

[15]See D N Saraf, Law of Consumer Protection in India 209, 2nd ed (1995) N.M.Tripathi Pvt Ltd, Mumbai.

[16]Common Cause v Union of India and others with Consumer Education and Research Society v Union of India, AIR 1993 SC 1403.

1975. Different yardsticks were made applicable to traders, professionals and those engaged in other vocations and the levies and applicable modes for evaluating the liability of each of the classes were also distinct.

Analysis:'Consumer', 'Service', 'Deficiency'

Under section 2(1)(d) of the CPA,[17] as amended in 1993, the term 'consumer' has been specifically defined in two parts: the first part refers to "buyer of goods for consideration," a phraseology which has, by and large, not created any interpretational problems, and the second, to "hiring or availing of any services for consideration" which has been the focus of judicial interpretation, leading to the widening of the scope of application of CPA by reading the terms and provisions with hair-splitting interpretations. The term 'services' was initially defined to mean "service of any description which is made available to potential users, and includes in its provisions numerous enlisted facilities like banking, financing, insurance, etc." but excludes the "rendering of any service free of charge or under a contract of personal service."[18] The service of "housing construction" was later included by the Amending Act of 1993. Medical services per se still do not find any placement in the specific list.

The definition of 'services' itself enlists more than ten different ventures and invariably all of them contain one specific trend or norm, a single thread conspicuously running through each one of them, which is, 'commerce' engaged in by business houses and the like. Though it cannot be said or argued that the definition is exhaustive and therefore no venture, not specifically mentioned,[19]

---

[17]See Appendix A-Part C.

[18]S. 2(1)(o) Consumer Protection Act, 1986: Appendix A-Part C.

[19]Those included by specific mention in the definition of service are: banking, financing, insurance, transport, processing, supply of electricity or other energy board or lodging or both, housing construction, entertainment, amusement or the purveying of news of other information.

can be read into the Act as included, yet for determining whether a particular venture is included or not, application of the general principle of eugesdem generis* would be an important test.

Let us consider the example of a bank or an insurance company. Primarily a business venture, a bank offers its expert services to clients who in turn hire them for collecting and depositing their monies, making payments against cheques issued by them, and finally paying them interest on the deposits retained with the bank. The aims and objects underlying a bank offering services are to engage in commerce and make profits, which, if it is a public limited company, would be distributed amongst the shareholders.

In the case of an insurance company,[20] again a big business house, the offer is of covering insurable risks against payment of premiums so that the insurance company can use the monies so collected in commerce, make money and then, at the stipulated time, to hand over the assured sum with or without profits as the policy may stipulate, to the insured.

The basic idea is to utilise the monies, obtained against services that are offered, in money making ventures, make overall profits and after deducting the cost incurred in fulfilling the hire terms, to pass on a portion thereof to the hirer of services by way of interest or insurance cover, as the case may be. These are

*See Glossary.

[20]For example, The State Bank of India which has declared huge profits for the year 1995-96 a part of which will be distributed to shareholders by way of dividend. Likewise, The Unit Trust of India, a financing institution, engages a battery of experts in finance and offers their expertise as services to the public with a view of making big money. It comes out with tempting investment offers and has a large number of investor-clients as a huge scheme of commercialisation of finance-management services. The General Insurance company, a heavy profit making company which pays off the endowment or life security pay-offs along with bonuses against premiums paid by the insured. The Maharashtra State Road Transport Corporation is another commercial venture which offers transport services to a large number of commuters by running a huge fleet of public buses and earns huge profits out of the venture.

undisputedly the underlying aims and objects of the ventures in both cases. So is the case with each and every venture enlisted in the definition.

The legislation protects the rights of consumers who hire services of the class specified under the Act, while at the same time, services rendered free of charge or under a contract of personal service, have been specifically excluded from its purview. The consumers who utilise or hire services and who have a complaint against the service rendered come before the consumer forums for redressal of their grievances and are compensated by way of damages if the services are found to have suffered from 'deficiency' within the meaning of section 2(1)(g)[21] of the Act. The term 'deficiency' has been defined in the broadest possible terms to mean "any fault, imperfection, shortcoming or inadequacy in the quality, nature and manner of performance...."[22] Whereas the defect in the goods supplied may be rectifiable, or the goods themselves capable of being replaced or repaired, the deficiency in the services can be compensated by award of a just equivalent of the value or damages for the loss incurred. In either case, it does appear that the deficiency is capable of being determined in terms of money so as to compensate the defect or the loss.

Does the medical man fit into this picture? In the first place, the principle of 'buyer beware', a corollary to expert marketing strategies, never extended to the field of medicine which was based on mutual trust between a doctor and the patient. Whereas a trader, manufacturer, civil contractor or builder were all dealing with goods and could offer guarantee of their expertise in production and compensation in terms of monetary loss can be fixed, a doctor handling human lives could guarantee no success in his endeavour to aid human being in suffering nor is it possible to suggest an equivalent for suffering in terms of money. It is not in the medico's

[21]See Appendix A-Part C.

[22]*Ibid.*

hands to nullify the risk attached to every life, at every stage, at every moment, by quality control as can be done to achieve excellence in production. Neither guarantee nor warranty of the human body nor any part thereof can be given by the one whose services are said to be 'hired.' No money equivalent for loss of life or limb can exist.

The Supreme Court Contribution

On 13 November 1995, nearly a decade after the enforcement of CPA, a three member bench of the Supreme Court of India had, by their judgment in *Indian Medical Association v V P Shantha,*[23] struck a final seal on the long standing debate, extending, by judicial interpretation, the application of the CPA to members of the medical profession. The judgment places professionals within the network of legislation, factually, literally and primarily intended to protect the innocent consumers[24] from the malpractices of the menacing traders, encouraging ethical conduct in those engaged in the production and distribution of goods and rendering services to consumers,[25] a socio-economic legislation with a fundamental thrust on speedy redressal and monetary compensation. The doctors had for long hoped, albeit in vain, that the highest court would read the statute as it stood and not club them in the legislation apparently meant for commercial ventures and thus salvage the faith-abiding doctor-patient relationship of times immemorial.

Various distinctions which militate against the clamping of

---

[23]*Supra* n 5.

[24]*Supra* n 14.

[25]The General Assembly of the United Nations by Consumer Protection Resolution No: 39/248 adopted guidelines towards framing, for governments, particularly those of developing countries, to use in elaborating and strengthening consumer protection policies and legislation. The objectives of the said guidelines include assisting countries in achieving or maintaining adequate protection for their population as consumers and encouraging high levels of ethical conduct for those engaged in the production and distribution of goods and services to the consumers.

the Act on the doctors include:

- while a person engaged in an occupation renders service in the stream of commerce which is an essential ingredient for liability under the Act, the services rendered by a person belonging to a profession, bereft of any commercial ingredients, cannot fall within its ambit;
- medical practitioners were already governed by the provisions of the Indian Medical Council Act, 1956, and the code of medical ethics,[26] made by the Medical Council of India as approved by the Government of India under Section 3 of the Indian Medical Council Act, 1956, which regulates their conduct as members of the medical profession and provides for disciplinary action against a person for professional misconduct by the Medical Council of India and /or State Medical Councils and, therefore, no exigencies demanded an additional avenue for redressal;
- the use of expression "which is made available to potential users" contained in section 2(1)(o) of the Act (which defines 'service'), itself militates against the views that medical practitioners were contemplated by the Parliament to be covered within the provisions of the Act;
- the said expression indicates the kind of service the statute contemplates, namely, service of an institutional type which is a commercial enterprise and open and available to all who seek to avail there of;
- the definition of 'deficiency' which, under the Act means, "any fault, imperfection, short coming or inadequacy" in respect of a service, has to be ascertained on the basis of certain norms relating to quality, nature and manner of performance and the

[26] As approved by the Government of India under section 3 of the Indian Medical Council Act, 1956.

resultant produce, whereas, medical services rendered by a medical practitioner cannot be adjudged on the basis of any fixed norms;

- that composition of the District Forums, the State Commissions and the National Commission, all seem to militate against such inclusion as none is included who could fully appreciate the medical complexities;
- that the procedure that is followed by these bodies for determination of issues before them is not conducive for determination of the complicated questions which arise in respect of claims for medical negligence;
- that the relationship between the medical practitioner and the patient is of faith and confidence and, therefore, it is in the nature of a contract of personal service and the service rendered by the medical practitioner to the patient is not 'service' under section 2(1)(o) of the Act; However, while negativing the arguments put forth before the Supreme Court, on behalf of the medical practitioners, their Lordships observed that:
- the term 'profession' involves the idea of an occupation requiring either intellectual skill, or manual skill controlled, as in painting and sculpture,[27] or surgery, by the intellectual skill of the operator, as distinguished from an occupation which is substantially the production or sale or arrangement for the production or sale of commodities;[28]

---

[27]However, the examples cited by the court, i.e.painter and sculptor are both of the variety which produce 'goods' unlike surgeons who do not produce anything out of their skill. Hence, the comparison appears ill-fitting.

[28]Relying on Rupert M. Jackson and John L. Powell, Professional Negligence, 3rd ed, Their Lordships explained that the occupations which are regarded as professions have four characteristics, viz.,
i) the nature of the work which is skilled and specialized and a substantial part is mental rather than manual;
ii) commitment to moral principles which go beyond the general duty of honesty and a wider duty to community which may transcend the duty to a particular client or patient;
iii) professional association which regulates admission and seeks to uphold the standards of the profession through professional codes on matters of conduct and ethics; and
iv) high status in the community.

- the fact that they are governed by the Indian Medical Council Act and are subject to the disciplinary control of Medical Council of India and /or State Medical Councils is no solace to the person who has suffered due to their negligence and the right of such person to seek redress is not affected;
- from the use of the word 'potential users' it cannot be inferred that the service by medical practitioners are not contemplated by Parliament to be covered within the expression 'service' as contained in section 2(1)(o);
- section 14(1)(d) would indicate that the compensation to be awarded is for loss or injury suffered by the consumer due to the negligence of the opposite party. A determination of deficiency in service for the purpose of section 2(1)(g) has therefore to be made by applying the same test as is applied in an action for damages for negligence;
- since the goods or services in respect of which a complaint can be filed under the Act may relate to number of fields, it cannot be expected that the members of the Consumer Disputes Redressal Agencies must have expertise in the field to which the goods or services, in respect of which complaint is filed, are related. It will be for the parties to place the necessary material and the knowledge and experience which the members will have in the fields indicated in the Act would enable them to arrive at their findings on the basis of that material;
- in complaints involving complicated issues requiring recording of evidence of experts, the complainant can be asked to approach the Civil Court for appropriate relief. Section 3 of the Act which prescribes that the provisions of the Act shall be in addition to and not in derogation of the provisions of any other law for the time being in force, preserves the right of the consumer to approach the Civil Court for necessary relief;

- the relationship between the medical practitioner and the patient carries within it certain degree of mutual faith, confidence and trust and, therefore, the services rendered by the medical practitoner can be regarded as service of personal nature but since there is no relationship of master and servant between the doctor and his patient, the contract between the medical practitioner and his patient cannot be treated as a contract of personal service but is a contract for services and service rendered by the medical practitioner to his patient under such a contract is not covered by the exclusionary part of the definition of 'service' contained in section 2(1)(o) of the Act.

Scope of Decision

The crux of the final verdict as contained in the judgment is that the CPA:

Includes:

- service rendered to a patient by a medical practitioner by way of consultation, diagnosis and treatment - both medicinal and surgical, as they are in the nature of a contract 'for' personal service and not 'of' personal service;
- service rendered by a medical officer in employment, to an employee, is a 'contract of personal service;'
- services rendered at a non-governmental hospital / nursing home where charges are required to be paid by persons availing such services; services rendered at a non-government hospital / nursing home where charges are required to be paid by some and not others;
- service rendered by a medical practitioner or hospital/nursing home, where the person availing service is covered by an insurance policy for medical care;
- service rendered by the above, where, under conditions of

service, the employer bears the expenses of medical treatment of an employee and his family members dependent on him.

Excludes:

- service rendered free of charge by a medical practitioner attached to a hospital or a nursing home, or a medical officer employed in a hospital or nursing home where such services are rendered free to one and all;
- service rendered at a non-government hospital or nursing home where no charge whatsoever is made from any person availing the service;
- service rendered at a government hospital or a health centre dispensary where no charge whatsoever is taken from any person.

A few significant querries arise:

- did the Parliament consider life so worthless or the socialistic pattern of society so flimsy as to bar the poor and the needy from this supposedly easy, cheap and quick method of redressal?
- is it only or mainly the affluent who are the victims of deficient services of attending doctors or, are the free patients, treated like 'no class citizens' in the hospitals, the real sufferers?
- is there any logic in permitting this sacrilege on the poor in an avowed socialistic pattern of society? Or is it that they have the wherewithal for knocking at the doors of civil and criminal forums which the affluent do not possess?
- did the Parliament consider the professionals less important than the traders and the agriculturists so as to leave the supervisory jurisdiction in the hands of Minister for Agriculture and not the Minister for Health or Law?
- was the Parliament so unconcerned about the sick and the diseased or uninformed of the complexities of medical

knowledge that while framing a Council of Advisors consisting of 150 members, which include farmers, social workers etc, not one member from the medical profession was thought necessary in the configuration?

Analysis vis-a-vis Doctors

Factually, none of the definitions, provisions and set-up under the Act, as it came into force in 1986, even remotely refer to the medical, the legal or any other profession.

The Act as enacted, starting from the very aims and objects underlying the legislation, to the definitions, the provisions, the set-up of the Redressal Forums and Councils, right upto the supervisory administrative heads, does not once refer to the whole lot of important fraternities of professionals or make a specific mention that any professional was intended to be brought under its net. The absence of this intention is more than evident from various other provisions too. A Central Council consisting of 150 members[29] including ministers, members of parliament and other representatives of consumer organisations, farmers, trade and industries, social workers, women etc. is prescribed but none to represent this vast medical fraternity which has to work, day and

---

[29] (a) the Minister-in-charge of Department of Civil Supplies who shall be the Chairman of the Central Council; (b) the Minister of State (where he is not holding independent charge) or Deputy Minister in the Department of Civil Supplies who shall be the Vice-Chairman of the Central Council; (c) the Ministers of Food and Civil Supplies or Minister-in-Charge of Consumer Affairs in States; (d) eight Members of Parliament - five from the Lok Sabha and three from the Rajya Sabha; (e) the Commissioner for Scheduled Castes and Scheduled Tribes; (f) representatives of the Central Government Departments' autonomous organisations concerned with consumer interests - not exceeding twenty; (g) representatives of the Consumer Organisations for consumers not less than thirty-five; (h) representatives of women - not less than ten; (i) representatives of farmers, trade and industries — not exceeding twenty; (j) persons capable of representing consumer interests not specified above - not exceeding fifteen; (k) the Secretary in the Department of Civil Supplies shall be the member-secretary of the Central Council.

night, for the benefit of human life. Even the legal professional has a safeguard as a judge to head the forum, who is surely an expert in laws, but not the doctor. And the worst part is that the Act is eloquently silent, with a self-speaking clarity, with the total absence of the words 'medical treatment' or 'doctor' or 'profession' or 'patient', that there never was an intention on the part of the legislators to cover doctors and their services under the umbrella of the CPA. This must have been the reason why years had to elapse before a case was filed before the Redressal Forum against a doctor and it required protracted arguments right upto the stage of Supreme Court to get at the interpretation that the Act did take in the professionals. It is an inclusion by interpretation that has left them in a worse position than if the Act had been passed with an avowed intention to cover them, giving due consideration to the community at every stage right from framing the aims and objects upto giving of representation in every forum, absence of which has harmed them and thrown them into a dead lane.

It needs to be emphasised that even the amendment made in 1993 has failed to touch this burning topic in spite of noisy challenges. In legal parlance, whenever hectic debates and presumptions are raised for application or otherwise of penal provisions, the legislators do step in to clear the doubts by means of amendments. Although amendment of the Act was in the offing and was actually introduced covering 'housing construction', which incidentally does fall within commerce and satisfies the principle of eugesdem generis compared with the ten ventures already listed, the medical professionals were just not referred to.

If the Parliament had intended to club profession with trade and commerce, within the network of the CPA, it was duty bound to be more specific and say so in clear terms right from the stage of aims and objects, definitions, etc. Was it that the Parliamentarians did not consider the doctor-patient disputes, howsoever few and far between, worth a specific mention? Or, is it more obviously the reverse that they had not intended to bring in this entire lot of medicos and patients, advocates and litigants and other professionals and their clients (non-commercial ventures) within this commerce linked statute? Had they intended this inclusion, surely there would have been some indication of a debate or a mention in the aims and objects and of course the legislation itself. Why should it have been left vaguely to interpretation by the judiciary by long years of indeterminate litigation to let this distinguished class know of their liability under the Act?

The definitions of 'consumer' read with 'service' and 'deficiency' in the Act are the ones which are of significance vis-a-vis the doctor, since the courts have, by and large, referred to 'medical services' as 'hired services' and the 'patient' as the 'consumer-cum-hirer' of the doctor's services. In the instant case, with due respect, analysing a few clauses in an attempt to fit in the professionals into the glove, for example, saying that a patient is a person who hires the doctor's services for consideration which has been paid or promised, in full or in part, or one who hires any services under any system of deferred payment, or any beneficiary of such services which have been hired as above with the approval of the person hiring the services, is not enough. It would be essential to further prove that the services hired are by persons as defined in the term 'service' read in the light of the ten or more instances mentioned; that the basic purpose of the one offering services is commerce and so on.

It would appear that for a medical person to fit into the provisions of the Act, he must fall in line with the enlisted ventures, i.e. he must be one to offer his services for purposeful gains in the stream of commerce, and the patient, a consumer, must hire the doctor's services for obtaining gains out of the commercial venture of the one whose services he has hired, i.e. the doctor. Factually, commerce is not the base root of medical treatment. In a doctor-patient equation, for the doctor, serving the sick and diseased humanity must supercede all other considerations and the fees or compensation paid to the doctor only incidental to the main objective which is to cure, provide relief, or at least comfort the patient as far and as much as possible.

A close analysis brings to light a marked difference between a normal business and/or commercial venture offering services on hire and medical services. A seller, a producer, a manufacturer, are a class which produce goods for consumption (or use), while a person or business house which offers only services on hire do so for taking monies for use in ventures bringing material gains and then returning the monies at pre-determined intervals, or on demand, so on and so forth, both the hirer and the hired gaining materially from the transaction of service. Does the glove fit the medical hand?

Likewise, in services, one knows clearly what gains to expect, for, it is commerce that lies in between the hirer and the hired. In any case, a doctor is perfectly at liberty to charge the professional fees which he deems fit.[30] At the same time, the impossibility of guarantee of the outcome of a doctor's treatment and the patient's knowledge that the doctor is merely trying his best to comfort, if not cure him, is enough to demarcate the services envisaged by the legislators while drafting or passing the CPA from those rendered by a medical man. With due respect to the judicial pronouncement, this one distinct demarcation in itself is sufficient to clinch the whole issue. The absence of the pivotal commercial element in the patient's act of paying the treatment charges and the doctor accepting his professional fees for having treated a patient, militate against the very pronouncement that the Act was intended to or has unwittingly used the language due to which the medical

[30] In B.S. Hegde v. Dr. Sudhansu Bhattacharya, 1993(3) CPR 414 (NCDRC) the National Commission held that: "however improper it may be, the demand and acceptance of an exorbitant fee cannot be deemed to be deficiency in service and hence it is not for the consumer forums to adjudicate on the question whether the consideration charged was reasonable."

fraternity could be swept into the clutches of the Act.

Distinction between compensation for 'deficiency in services' by a commercial venture and that of a medico, are also significant. When services of a doctor are deficient, they can lead to loss of life or limb and surely human life or suffering cannot be evaluated or compensated in terms of monetary consideration, whatever be the amount. Thus, no fixed norms can be prescribed even by courts in case of their conclusion of deficiency in services by a medical man. In fact, the gap in expectation and award in the few cases decided has been phenomenal.

The yardstick is absolutely fluid, with no parameters whatsoever. In a matter before the National Commission, a lady was operated upon under general anaesthesia for delivery of a child by Cesarean section. Severe abdominal pain and nausea necessitated repeat surgery. The relatives were informed that about three feet of dead intestine material had to be resected; which would be a difficult process as swelling of the intestine and oedematous tissue had already set in. During surgery, however, an artery forceps was found entwined in the intestinal material removed. It was this foreign invasion which had apparently obstructed the blood supply to the intestine, resulting in repeat operation, followed by gangrene. The compensation claimed by the parties (besides expenses) was Rs 8,50,000/- against which a mere pittance of Rs 2000/- was sanctioned by the State Commission which was subsequently raised by the National Commission to 10,000/-.[31] Was anything gained by the sufferer by the introduction of the newly created forum, the Consumer Forum vis-a-vis the Civil Court?

Moreover, the very essence of medical practice is such that no hard and fast rules can apply in diagnosis and treatment. Barring those cases where negligence is evident on the face of it, like where a gauze towel was left in the abdominal cavity necessitating re-

[31]Sau. Madhuri v Dr Rajendra, (1996) III CPJ 75, at 76 (NC).

operation for removal and consequent post-splenectomy fever and septicaemia,[32] or where a person qualified in homeopathy practices allopathy,[33] or failure to attend to calls after accepting the responsibility of the patient, or a surgeon not attending personally to the operation, or a hospital not being adequately equipped to handle the cases it accepts are the apparent cases which speak for themselves (*res ipsa loquiyter*), by and large, the entire project is most subjective and individualised and, more often than not, differs from individual to individual medico. Thus in every case of a complaint also, the main criterion for determining existence or non-existence of deficiency in services, would be whether the doctor had exercised his skill and reasonable care in the performance of his medical duties or had failed to do so in some way. The 'reasonableness' of skill and care required is again a variable, depending on the circumstances of each individual case.

Another important factor, which militates against the judicial pronouncement is violating the very basics of an avowed socialistic pattern of society, relates to 'free services.' As *per* the judgment, in specified cases at least, if there is no consideration, there can be no hiring of services and therefore, in any case, free beneficiaries of services are out of the purview of the Act. Only those patients who pay the fees can have access to Consumer Forums. Every litigant has to produce satisfactory evidence of payment made to the doctor or the hospital to be categorised as a 'consumer.' In a socialistic pattern of society, is this not a discrimination not based on any rationale?

Yet, it is in this context that the Supreme Court has been constrained to hold that even though medical men fall within the ambit of the Act, their services being hired in the sense that they

[32]*Ramanand B. Raikar v Salgaonkar Medical Research Centre and another*, 1993 (3) CPR 300.

[33]*Poonam Verma v Ashwin Patel and others*, AIR 1996 SC 2111.

are for consideration, those medical professionals, government hospitals, nursing homes and private hospitals or where "services are rendered free of charge to every patient are excluded from the purview of the Act."[34] The Supreme Court has been cautious enough not to exclude even those hospitals where charges are required to be paid by persons availing services "except certain categories of persons who cannot afford to pay and are thus rendered free service." In preferring this far-fetched, discriminatory and anti-socialistic interpretation of the Act, the court has by-passed the basic pillar of commercial gains obtained or intended to be obtained by the supplier of goods or the one who offers services on hire or the one who hires services of another.

In a case, a lady underwent an operation for the removal of gall bladder and died. The claim of compensation put forth by the survivors was opposed on the ground that the operation was performed gratuitous as the brother of the deceased was a family friend of the doctor working in the same hospital. The complainant however insisted that he had paid Rs. 3500/- instead of Rs.7,000/- that were demanded but was unable to produce proof of payment. This lacuna in evidence proved fatal to the charge made out by the complainant and the petition was dismissed.[35] Is the decision towing the socialistic pattern of society, or indeed, imparting justice to the aggrieved?

An interesting case on this point came before the Maharashtra State Consumer Disputes Redressal Commission.[36] Smt. Sunita, a woman with a cardiac complaint, was admitted to Miraj Medical Centre, Wanless Hospital, Miraj and operated upon. Consequent to administration of blood by the hospital, she contracted AIDS. It was alleged that subsequently, even her husband and the small child born after surgery, had got afflicted with the virus. A claim

---

[34] *Supra* n 5.

[35] *S.S. Kahlon & Anr v. Bawa Hospital*, 1994 (1) CPR 773 (SCDRC, Punjab).

[36] *Sau Sunita Vasant Heganawar v. Miraj Medical Centre*, II (1994) CPJ 544.

for rupees ten lacs was put forth before the Forum. Despite the hospital having admitted administering HIV+ blood, without testing, in view of emergency, the petition failed on the ground that Miraj Medical Centre was a charitable hospital run by the Christian Mission and that "the treatment given to the complainant was free of charge."

Thus, if indeed the medical services are covered by the Act, it is a sad reflection on the legislators that they permitted this sacrilege of the masses inasmuch as, professionals and hospitals rendering services free, escape the clutches of accountability under the cheap, supposedly speedy and informal forum of redressal and, to that extent, are permitted to go on harming the masses to any extent. In fact, the consumer activists have oftentimes argued that the taxes paid to the government go into funding of hospitals run by States out of which the medical staff is paid salaries, and, therefore, although they do not charge the individual patient they do receive consideration for the services offered to patients. Hence, there is no reason for excluding them from the purview of the Act even by interpretation.

While one can understand the logic behind free services rendered for production of goods or otherwise, being excluded from liability to pay compensation to the hirer, the very notion militates against treating human lives on par with goods so that even if a human life or limb is lost, the sufferers should by law be excluded from claiming compensation under the Act only on the premise that the patient had been treated free of charge. The very idea is revolting in a democratic state with avowed socialistic pattern of society and hits one in the eye.

A reading of the judgment of the Supreme Court leaves one with the indisputable impression that the decision rests on the basis that the Act ought to have covered the services rendered by doctors as is done in countries abroad rather than whether factually it did cover them or not. Relying on a battery of foreign authorities and case laws,[37] it has gone more by their opinion that consumerism laws abroad having covered the professionals, the CPA can and ought to be read as covering them in India too. However, the basic differences in the health laws in England, the fact that the National Health Scheme regulates the work of panel doctors and in the United States of America where different considerations prevail in treatment of patients in hospitals and the super specialists called in for attending to complications, were neither considered nor discussed while extending the legal dicta of other countries to legal conclusions in India. The judgment hardly answers the question: did the legislation intend to or even as passed, clearly and unambiguously cover the professional and if so, why were the entire battery of terminology of professionals, patients, litigants, medical and legal services left out from the vocabulary used and then why would only the medical profession have been segregated from farmers, social workers, women representatives etc, by not giving them even one representative in the Consumer Council?

For ages, trade and profession have been distinguished, trade being corelated to sale of goods and the like, or services offered for production with commercial gains being the main basis. 'Profession' is distinguished from `trade' and `occupation' by (a) specialised training and certification; (b) peer group accountability and self regulation; (c) consideration of public service or good in ways that trade, occupation, business may not or need not be. The doctors

---

[37]Those referred to are : Rupert M Jackson and John L Powell, *Professional Negligence* 3rd ed; Mason & Mc Call Smith, *Law and Medical Ethics* 4th ed; *Commissioners of Inland Revenue v Maxse* (1919) 1 KB 647, 657; *Saif Ali v Sidney Mitchell & Co* (1980) 1 AC 198; *Rees v Sinclair* (1974) 1 NZLR 180; *Giaannarelli v Wrath* (1988) 81 ALR 417; *Arizona v Maricopa County Medical Society* 457 US 332; *Bolam v Friern Hospital Management Committee* (1957) 1WLR 582; *Whitehouse v Jordan* (1981) (1) WLR 246; *Maynard v West Midlands Regional Health Authority* 1984 (1) WLR 634; *Sidaway v Governors of Bethlem Royal Hospital*, 1985 AC 871; *Simmons v Health Laundry Co* (1910) 1 KB 543; *Whitehouse v Jordan & Anr* (1980) 1 All ER 650.

unequivocal stand has been that they offer services to patients and not consumers, that their services are not hired but are placed at the disposal of the sick for serving humanity and that they are enriching human lives and not manufacturing or selling and supplying or even handling goods which can be covered by guarantees or warrantees against defects or wherein defects can be compensated by money or replacement.

Implications

It is true that the wave of judicial activism, or may be, creativism, itself was born of noble endeavours, apparently, that of coming to the aid of the masses, at a time when the entire citizenry stood frustrated and their hopes reduced to naught by the turn the national polity had taken with corruption and criminalisation polluting the sacred portals. However, whether the liberalised interpretation to placate the medical fraternity, has and is going to benefit the masses or not, needs proper evaluation.

It needs to be highlighted that it was not as if by this decision, the accountability of doctors had been newly created or enhanced, for they had always been accountable under their long-existing self regulatory recognised codes, as well as the civil and criminal laws under which they were punishable since the very inception of the respective codes. Factually, the patient has and had always enjoyed a right to his doctor's correct, conscientious, diligent and skilled services and doctors have always been, and continue to be, notwithstanding the CPA, liable for damages under civil laws (tort), and for punishment for medical negligence under criminal laws. For example, a doctor is and has been liable for imprisonment upto two years or fine or both under section 304A of The Indian Penal Code, 1860, for death caused by his "rash and negligent act." Likewise, a hospital has been and continues to be vicariously liable, under civil laws, for the negligence of doctors and the technical staff working there. Such liability has existed since the days of onset of civil and criminal liabilities under Roman law, and have been formally launched with the enforcement of the codified laws. No doctor or a medical representative body has ever questioned the accountability of their members or the provisions for punishment under the laws. Nor have they ever been shown any laxity in case of a negligent act. Even with the decision of the Apex Court, the liability under the various laws has remained intact. The CPA is just an additional legal avenue for their prosecution and professes to have been enacted to ensure an almost free and speedy redressal to consumers,[38] in this case the patients, without strict observance of the procedures, rules and norms which govern court trials and without intervention of lawyers whose allegedly high fees the individual litigants may not be able to afford. It has, however, unfortunately though, come to be looked upon by the consumers as an easy forum to vent their grievances, at times impulsive and born out of acute emotions aroused momentarily, by calamitous circumstances or even in the hope of making a quick buck and, in any case, losing nothing.

Yet, no amount of consolation that the addition is merely a new avenue already encountering the 'delay syndrome' seems to offer any succour to the disgruntled lot. Known for their expertise at curing human beings, their skills in mending limbs, their years of prolonged efforts at providing succour to the suffering patients at all odd hours of the day and night, their attempts to improve the quality of life or prolong life span by risk involving surgeries including organ transplants, the doctors today look askance at the law lords, their debates soon turning into fire and smoke when it comes to the CPA wherein they find their skillful services clubbed with trade

---

[38]The professed guarantee of speedy redressal in the litigation under the Act has already been belied as a myth. "By its utter neglect of State Consumer Courts, the Maharashtra Government has forfeited a huge Central grant meant for the disposal of pending cases in these courts.... currently there is a backlog of nearly 5,000 cases in the State Commission alone. Statewide, the pendency figure is over 33,000.": See, *The Daily* (Bombay ed) 7 December 1996.

and commerce, not by the Parliament, but, according to them, by interpretation of the provisions of the Act by the judiciary during a period when judicial activism was at its peak.

Unfortunately, the spontaneous outcome of this decision has been a feeling of insecurity amongst the doctors derived from the very apprehension of being dragged into a net not befitting or appropriate to their profession even in rarest of rare cases. In search of ways to reduce risks inevitable in the very nature of their work and in a bid to share or transfer the burden of their accountability and diffuse the liability, in case of any mishap, a buffer system of a whole gamut of expensive investigations have cropped up almost overnight.[39] Leave aside complicated cases, even simple fevers normally dealt with by the well experienced family physician, are now being processed through the pathologist, the radiologist, the sonologist, the .....gist or may be even the astrologer. Even dentists have started insisting on blood, bowel and ECG reports before filling cavities under local anaesthesia. Sophisticated investigations, blood report, HIV factor, chest X-Ray, Magnetic Resonance Imaging, sonography, etc have suddenly been introduced "in the interest of the patient." Complex and costly conglomerate references, in most cases beyond the capacity of the average affording individual, has taken over the direct doctor-patient equation. In many cases, the patients are directed or rather accompanied to the consultant and then the consultant's consultant, or the super specialist, before prescribing the treatment. In foreign countries, such procedures are the accepted norms and medical expenses covered by insurance but what about a country like ours where poverty abounds? The patients are now made to go round and round from pillar to post for getting diagnosis related reports, making medical treatment an enormous economic burden on the already suffering sick.

What about the doctors? Whereas the corporate bigwigs who

[39]For details, see: Appendix C.

get enmeshed in economic crimes can, through their business channels, pay the formidable cost of litigation and/or compensation or damages, for doctors litigation is a nightmare. Even a false and frivolous complaint is, for them, fatal to their practice, prestige and popularity. With one stroke, the reputation built, bit by bit, brick by brick, on the rock foundation of specialised training of long years, hard work, goodwill and acquired skill which had carried them off to the peak of success, comes tumbling down like a pack of cards. Many a successful doctor has developed a feeling of just wanting to escape from it all rather than go on facing degrading trials and fall into the network of law, attempting to brief the anatomy illiterate lawyers and to convince the bench, with complete lack of knowledge of medical intricacies and saddled with the objective of speedy disposal, of their skilled services.

Another outcome which roused its head just as the first whispers of the judgment became audible was that many doctors took the professional insurance cover and the insurance companies quickly rose to make hay while the sun shines, marketing their policies, aiming at an immediate business involving big monies from the doctors, the vulnerable victims, only too willing to take the 'cover,' following a compulsive system which has been rampant abroad for over two or three decades. They struck the coveted bargain.[40] However, almost immediately, the risk coverage expenses incurred by them were passed on to the 'consumers' of their 'hired' medical services.

Is it surprising then that there has been a sudden spurt in medical expenses that the sick have had to bear, for not only do the patients have to undergo a tremendous volley of investigations for the safety of the doctor before he, the doctor, will even venture into actual medication? All the same, they have to, albeit indirectly, shell out part of the heavy insurance coverage for the doctors too.

---

[40]*Ibid.*

More and more doctors have begun to refuse emergency cases, more and more have started charging under the table to take shelter under free treatment clause and it is the genuine patients who are running helter skelter hunting for the old nobility amongst the medical profession.

One may as well ask: is the repercussion justified? There is a long standing natural tendency of the patients and their near ones to expect the doctor to perform miracles and overcome any eventuality or even the ultimate calamity. When emotions vibe on high frequencies, they could pave a pathway to innumerable inappropriate litigations at the hands of those who think they or their near ones could have been saved but were not. After all it cannot be gainsaid that in times of emergencies or when the end is near, or when the patient is in acute pain, the dear ones of the sick are insatiable when it comes to the requirement of the doctor's time and attention. Or, may be, a few litigations will come up at the hands of others wanting to settle various scores or even by a few at the instigation of competing doctors as, in any case, neither have two lawyers ever agreed on the correct legalities, nor do two doctors think alike on remedies, given the same set of circumstances.

The easy pathway can thus prove to be a by-lane for false or frivolous litigation initiated by the distraught aggrieved. The professed safeguards against vexatious complaints are not at all effective redeeming factors for a doctor whose professional reputation is bound to be affected by a single complaint blown out of proportion by the press and the law reporters, whatever be its ultimate fate. To add to their grievances, the paramount judicial delays have already beseiged the consumer forums and the working of the forums appears to be in doldrums. It can now be surmised that the litigation once initiated against any individual doctor, who may have had the misfortune of being dragged into this forum, will last for an indefinite period, the time factor itself proving fatal to his practice.

What does the future hold for us as a nation? The acid test of 'benefit to the masses' by labelling patients as 'consumers,' must necessarily lie in the answer to the question: has or will the interpretation preferred by the Honorable judges indeed benefit the sick and needy masses of India? In such an environment, with the impractical and ill-conceived reservations in vogue, the high fees imposed even on merit students for entering the medical stream, the future wrought with more hurdles than ever before, the field will soon be devoid of those intellectual and noble souls who would have wished to enter the medical field to serve humanity with all the vigour and gusto of entering a noble profession.

Alternative Solutions:

The Medical Council of India formed under the Indian Medical Council Act, 1956 with Government approval was created as a conduct and disciplinary code against the doctors just as the Bar Council of India was created for lawyers.[41] Even today, the Code of Medical Ethics framed by the Council regulates the conduct of the medical fraternity. The Medical Council, manned by those well versed in the science of medicine, had been voicing a demand for more penal powers to be able to act against the erring members effectively but their requests have fallen on deaf ears, their correspondence confined to the lowest drawers and their voice blown off into wilderness. Had the government acted in time to strengthen the Councils and clothed them with suitable powers, its functioning would have filled the void that was later felt and sort of filled by the interpretation of CPA. Had the lawyer advising the first test case patient to try out the Consuner Forum been conscious that by a far-fetched interpretation that medical services were hired services etc, he was thrusting not only the medical fraternity but also his brethren, the lawyers, into the legislation for trade and commerce, there would indeed have been no precedent

[41]See, *supra nos*: 3 and 4.

of the single disgruntled case attempting to get redress under a trader-consumer forum and not the forum governing such professionals. Indeed, the inaction of government and the complacency, nay, the ineffective demands by the medical fraternity coupled with the usual ingenuity of the lawyers to find out loop holes in law and fit in their cases rather than working towards streamlining of effective laws through judicial interpretations have together formed a multi edged weapon which has caused the judiciary to step in and take the profession by the horns presumably in public interest, in times when the seed of judicial activism had already sprouted into a fertile field.

Conclusion

Considering the environment all around, the economic poverty and the gross illiteracy of the nation, the need of medical men for the rural masses and the large brain drain caused by job satisfaction accompanied by exuberant earnings available to doctors abroad, the need of the hour is to knit a golden thread which should entwine the doctor and the patient in a cordial relationship of faith, compassion and confidence, weighing the services that a doctor can reasonably be expected to give to each patient under the circumstantial environment existing in the nation, rather than creating an unpalatable situation in the form of an inappropriate avenue which only has harmed the masses rather than aided them.

Factually, doctors form the top intelligentsia of the country. Undoubtedly, today, the order of merit for admissions goes as: medical, engineering and then law, commerce, etc. Unless working conditions are improved, the will of the youth to serve within the nation or even select medicine as a career is bound to be adversely affected. If the working conditions in the medical field are degrading, the temptation for doctors to migrate to greener pastures in countries looking out for medical men or even to divert from the medical field, will take over the youth of the nation with disastrous results.

The unwarranted reservations and quotas which have already infected the stream of education have created toxic fumes in the recent past and with the policy currently in vogue, the future will have to do with sub-standard doctors and surgeons and, inevitably, standard of services will go from bad to worse, deteriorating further and yet further. The nation is already facing a brain drain and such adverse conditions are bound to affect the medical aid in India to a staggering low.

The backlash will no doubt take a few years to highlight itself, for, in a country like India, the citizens have learnt to be complacent even to suffering till perhaps the disease cancerises the whole body as it has done in the politics of today and then some commissions will be formed to re-assess the situation, make recommendations and then there will be vociferous discussions in both Houses of Parliament, then a list of objections will be framed, then probably another high-power committee will be constituted and by the time the government takes a belated decision to make amends, objections notwithstanding, the government of the day will no longer be there and the subsequent party or a conglomeration forming government would undo everything and prefer to start afresh rather than implement the decisions by their predecessors. And thus the vicious circle will go on and on while the conditions go on deteriorating to the lowest levels of competency and the masses go on suffering. Years later, some changes may be thought necessary and a hurried legislation would be passed with loopholes galore and then the courts will take cognisance of the situation and justice may attempt to find its way out of the man-made rigmarole but get lost in the confusion. But by then, the harm would already have been done, thousands would have suffered avoidable mishaps.

The solution obviously cannot lie in enmeshing the professionals in a set-up that was specifically intended for trade and commerce. In any case, the statistics do not reveal any glorious benefi to the patients by the incorporation of these cases within the consumer net. The statistics from the National Consumer Disputes Redressal Forum, received while the book was going to print reveal: Total number of medical cases filed since 1989: 300(approx); Total number of medical cases disposed off till may 1998: 30 (approx); total number of medical cases decided against the doctors: 7. With the meagre disposal of cases involving doctors versus the great hype created one is given to think that need to take the erring doctors (and the lawyers) to task could very well be met by strengthening the provisions of the Medical Council of India[42] (and in the same vein, also the Bar Council of India) or framing a fresh legislation to deal with professionals by more clear-cut applicable statute and providing medical tribunals-cum-disciplinary committees at the central, state and district levels to look into complaints against doctors and hospitals, lawyers and other professionals.

Despite the final judicial word and the consumer activists projecting to the contrary, there are many valid arguments which could be outlined for releasing the medical fraternity from the tentacles of the CPA. An overview of the post-judgment situation leads one to the unstinted conclusion that the step has rather than improving medical aid in the country, adversely affected the life long doctor-patient faith-abiding relationship that had existed between families and their family doctors, a long standing aspect of the medical firmament in India, and hampered the spirit of service with which at least the majority of the doctors had been serving their patients till today, relying more on their clinical acumen than the battery of investigations. The fact that many doctors had hardly ever been conscious of the civil and criminal liabilities which have always existed is partly because doctors have been as ignorant of laws as lawyers of the human anatomy, and more so because doctors in India had always enjoyed utmost confidence of their patients

[42]For details, see: Appendix C.

and as it is, doctors, patients and their relatives are conscious of the risk that attends every medical treatment, with the result that only stray cases of frank medical negligence would have been installed against them.

As of today, the doctors feel that had they worked towards making the Indian Medical Association and its State branches strong enough to successfully resist this step-in avenue and moreso by having made the Association self-sufficient with powers which could have empowered it to adequately penalise its members, the doctors, the physicians and the surgeons, the neurologists and the oncologists, against bonafide sufferers through doctor's negligence, perhaps the extreme step of judicial intervention would not have materialised. Had the Association acted in time and honestly, without fear or favour, having been in existence for a sufficiently long period to have acquired teeth and created a strong legal avenue, the need for this liberalised activism for clamping an ill-fitting forum would not have arisen. It is perhaps the apparently innocuous existence of the Medical Associations and Bar Councils that has prompted judiciary or, before that, the consumer activists to have borrowed this extreme argument of consumerism inherent in medical services from foreign countries to gain justice for the sick.

However, the final attempt made by the IMA in the form of a review petition having failed to take off, a few viable alternatives can still be pursued. The IMA can think of approaching the Parliamentarians to amend the CPA to exclude the professionals notwithstanding the Courts decision which they can do coming out clearly with the factual aspect that the intention underlying the introduction of the statute was not to cover professions into the legislation which was primarily to safeguard malpractices in trade and commerce.

If the Parliament does desire to enact a fresh legislation to strealine professions against malpractices, medical or legal negligence etc., it can enact an appropriate legislation outside the purview of commercial ventures, taking the two main professions, the medical and legal, into confidence right from grass roots. Let the liability be specific and clear-cut and the avenue appropriate. In the alternative, let the government revamp the Medical and the Bar Councils and give them penal powers and appont suitable tribunals as in the case of government servants, motor accidents etc. to deal effectively with the two specific and other professions. An eloquent clarity in open seminars with regard to the ill effects that the clamping of CPA on doctors has had markedly on the sick and specially the emergency cases;[43] the phenomenal rise in the cost of medical treatment, could result in a strong case for the parliamentarians to consider enacting a separate legislation, outside the purview of 'consumerism,' to deal effectively with the medical fraternity considering the complexities and peculiarities of medical sciences.

Thus can positive results accrue, peace and goodwill restored between doctors and the patients, the activists and the needy masses, while achieving the goal of equality in medical facilities and avenues of redressal for the poor and the rich, the paying and the free patients, for all humanity must be dealt with alike before law, at least that is what the Constitution assures. The decision of the Apex Court clamping CPA on the doctors has, by means of the discrimination so spelt out, done more harm than good to the masses.

[43]For example, at The Annual National Conference of The Indian Orthopaedics Association held at Kochi in November 1997, the doctors flayed the growing harassment of doctors by Consumer Forums: See, The Afternoon, (Bombay ed) 1 December 1997.

Role of Consent in Medical Practice

Consent, one of the oldest conceptual aspects of law, an integral component in the contractual and criminal laws, plays a dominant role in human relations including the doctor-patient equation, may it be clinical practice or surgical intervention. The ethical principle of the right to self-determination is derived from the concept of consent. An otherwise actionable wrong raising a civil liability for damages or a crime calling for penal action, could be effectively assuaged under the blanket cover of 'consent.'

To what extent can the defence of 'consent' shield a doctor against liability? In which cases can it be used as an effective defence? These are the key issues which have gained immense importance for every medical man in his equation with patients. The simple act of obtaining a written consent of the patient, or the near relatives in case of a minor or a person of unsound mind or in an emergency case, before embarking on any surgery with its inevitable consequential risk, has been in practice since long.

Besides giving in brief a historical background of the concept of consent, the definition of the term under the law of contract and the criminal laws, as well as its scope in general and dealing with other co-related issues, this chapter highlights the significance of consent in medical practice. The manner and mode of obtaining it, circumstances whereunder a doctor's interests do acquire a protective umbrella against liability because of consent and cases wherein, under dire necessity, a doctor is protected even in the absence of an express consent are some of the aspects elaborated.

Historical Background

The origin of the concept of consent can be traced back to the days of early Greek[44] and Roman laws,[45] when life was deemed to belong to man as his self-owned property with unquestionable rights, when man had complete dominance on life and personal liberty of himself as well as his wife, children and slaves who were considered to be subjects of his private ownership, giving him exclusive powers to consent to any injury being caused or even to barter away their lives for mere pecuniary compensation. Consent came to acquire a wide sweep, a person being clothed with an unbridled power to consent to any injury of whatsoever nature and extent being caused to himself and his dependents.

With this backdrop, man had acquired an inherent right to determine the pattern of his life, even its expanse, or in other words whether and when to terminate it. Thus suicide was considered an inherent right of every 'free' man; the decision regarding mercy killing was left to his discretion; even murder could be committed with impunity -'might is right' was the predominant unwritten code of conduct. A human being could thus settle his grievances independent of laws and as *per* his might.

There arose a need to restrict the exercise of this crude and unmonitored right. Initially, the principle followed and what today is the basis of the retributive form of punishment was life for life, tooth for tooth, eye for eye, ensuring that harm caused by the assailant should be in equilibrium with that caused to him. This apparent, just and equitable retaliatory equation initiated, to monitor

---

[44]See Bury B, Cook S A, Adcock F E(ed), *The Cambridge Ancient History* 9 vol v (Athens 478-401) (1935) Cambridge University Press.

[45]Cook S A, F E Adcock, Charlesworth M P (ed), *The Cambridge Ancient History* 787, vol ix (The Roman Republic 133-44 B C) (1935) Cambridge University Press.

the harm caused and then to adjust and equate harm by the opponent forces, when emotions were bound to run high, proved to be a failure. Chaos and confusion prevailed for quite some time and then further deliberations ensued. Limitations and curbs were called for and their strict monitoring became inevitable. So developed the dictum *volenti non fit injuria.*[46]

The origin of this Latin maxim, popularly used in defence of situations where free citizens, at their will, sold themselves as slaves, dates back to the days of Aristotle. Later, adopted by the English common law in 1250 AD., by 1305 AD it was worded exactly the way it stands today.[47] The principles of equity, justice and good conscience are the underlying pillars of the maxim, based on the premise that man should not complain of harm to which he has consented with full knowledge and free will.

Some time later, with the development of the notion of society and the State, as *per* one school of thought, the latter could assert its rights and take up added responsibilities. On the one hand, the State gave unto itself the responsibility to protect every individual, and on the other, assumed the right to the lives of citizens as individuals. The entire notion of 'ownership' underwent a sea change. Every individual's life now belonged to the State. Thenceforth, no person had a right to take away his own life or to direct any other person to take it away. As a consequence, murder became penal, mercy killing was made punishable and attempt to commit suicide was made an offence. Even taking away the `life' of a foetus became a subject matter of legislation. The right to take away the life of an individual belonged only to the State and therefore capital punishment continued to figure in criminal laws and penal statutes. However, in turn, the State was cloaked with

---

[46]That is, damage suffered by consent is not a cause of action: Herbert Broom, *A Selection of Legal Maxims* 181, 10th ed (1995) Sweet & Maxwell, London.

[47]J.A.Jolowicz and T.Ellis Lewis (ed), *Winfield On Tort* 740, 8th ed (1967) Sweet & Maxwell, London.

the responsibility of maintaining law and order and securing the life of the citizens against external aggression during war or otherwise as well as against internal violation.

Consent

Consent, express or implied, is defined to mean "to agree to do something; to give one's permission for something"[48] or more commonly understood to mean concurrence of the will coupled with consciousness or comprehension of the act which is consented to. Consent means to concede or to concur; in other words, it means, "voluntary agreement, compliance or permission."[49] However, mere surrender to the will of another or submission, void of the element of voluntariness, would not amount to consent; that is, every consent involves submission but mere submission by no means amounts to consent.[50] A positive assertion of the mind is clearly distinguishable from mere submission, want of assent or acquiescence, although these may in certain situations constitute consent.

'Consent' finds its placement in civil as well as criminal laws. Under the civil forum, The Indian Contract Act, 1872 has dealt extensively with consent whereas under the criminal forum it is the Indian Penal Code, 1860 that deals with consent as understood in legal parlance.

Consent In Contract Law

Under the Indian Contract Act, consent is defined as two or more persons agreeing upon "the same thing in the same sense."[51] In the case of doctors and patients, 'the same thing' would mean

---

[48]*Chamber's 21st Century Dictionary* 291 (1997) Allied Chambers (India) Limited, New Delhi.

[49]Parikh, *Textbook of Medical Jurisprudence and Toxicology* 567, 5th ed (1990) CBS Publishers and Distributors.

[50]*Tukaram v State of Maharashtra,* AIR 1979 SC 185.

[51]S. 13 Indian Contract Act, 1872: See Appendix A-Part A.

the entire act of treatment, whether it consists wholly or in part of the giving of medical services, performance of surgery and/or payment of fees.

Consent, once it is given, can be revoked before the act consented to has commenced but not afterwards. Therefore, once a surgical procedure consented to has commenced, the surgeon would have a right to continue the operation until completion of the act consented to. Withdrawl of consent, midway, is not binding. Consent covers not only the act itself but also its natural consequences.

Section 14 of the Indian Contract Act, requires consent to be 'free' or not caused by coercion, undue influence, fraud, misrepresentation, mistake[52] (all the terms being understood as defined in the Act itself). Obviously, when coercion and the like have clouded the mind of the individual, not being free, consent lacks validity.

The key terms, 'coercion',[53] 'undue influence',[54] 'fraud',[55] 'misrepresentation,'[56] in the definition of contract as in the Indian Contract Act, have a significant bearing even in the doctor-patient equation. Coercion, in order to negative the validity of a contract, must be such so as to have operated on the mind of the person who has consented to the contract and it could be adjudged that the consent would not have been given but for the coercion irrespective of the quarter from which it had proceeded.

A contract is also invalidated if induced by 'undue influence,' the term 'influence' meaning 'power' of producing an effect. A person exercising such power, to exploit such an influence or

---

[52]See Appendix A-Part A.
[53]S. 15, *id.*
[54]S. 16, *id.*
[55]S. 17, *id.*
[56]S. 18, *id.*

authority in an unfair, unjustified, unmerited and unwarranted manner amounts to exercising 'undue influence.' Under the Indian Contract Act, a contract is said to be induced by undue influence, and therefore not free, if parties who are in a position to dominate the will of another, use their position to eclipse the mind of the other to thereby obtain unfair advantage over the other.

In effect, under the Contract Act, by an illustration, a contract can be negatived on the ground of 'undue influence' if one of the contracting parties, who stands in a fiduciary position* to the other, exercises a real or apparent authority over the other by either dominating the will and mind of the other or if such person is strong enough to dictate terms on one who is bound to depend upon him because of some mental infirmity or physical problem. Undue influence is also said to be exerted where the dominating parties have taken an undesirous benefit over the weaker party or the transaction is unconscionable.

The other factor which nullifies a contract is 'fraud,' whether committed by *suggestio falsi*, the suggestion of a false fact to the knowledge of the person making it; or by suppressio veri, the concealment of an essential fact. Either an attempt to deceive a person by a wilful act or to defraud another by purposeful silence and thereby inducing him to enter into an agreement which he would not have otherwise entered into, and is clearly to the detriment of his interest are instances of fraud.

Such a transaction, bearing its initial seed in false representation by one in order to induce another to act on that representation, to the advantage of the former and the disadvantage of the latter, is said to be 'fraudulent.' Section 17 of the Indian Contract Act describes the acts which could be labelled deceptive.[57] However, all attempts to define this complex feature have proved

---

*See Glossary.

[57] *Supra* n 55.

abortive, and the term is best understood by its concept.

Another factor which could negate a contract is 'misrepresentation' of essential facts. An unfounded positive communication of what is not true even though the person might believe it to be true; a breach of duty for the express purpose of misleading another to his own prejudice or that of anyone claiming under him; causing a party to a contract to make a mistake as to the subject matter of the agreement[58] are examples of misrepresentation.

The section defining the term opens with the words 'means and includes', making the definition an inclusive one which can, by the application of the principle of *ejusdem generis,** include within its fold several similar conditions. All these definitions under the Contract Act are illustrative, inclusive and not comprehensive.

Under section 19 of the Indian Contract Act, whenever consent to any agreement is obtained by coercion, fraud and/or misrepresentation, the agreement is a contract which is "voidable* at the option of the party whose consent was so caused."[59]

Consent in Criminal Law

The criminal law relating to consent contained in sections 87 to 92 of the Indian Penal Code,[60] basically revolves on the premise that a person can consent to any harm,* short of death or grievous hurt,* if the person is above twelve years of age. Apparently, consent forms a complete defence in such cases.

Thus, a person, above eighteen years of age can consent to suffer any harm, provided there is absence of intention* to cause death or grievous hurt or for an act not known by the doer to be likely to cause death or grievous hurt.[61] In fact, absence of intention

---

[58]Supra n 56.
*See Glossary. S. 19:
[59]See Appendix A-Part A.
[60]See Appendix A-Part B.
[61]S.87: See Appendix A-Part B.

to cause death can exempt a person from liability, whatever be the consequence of the act, provided the act was done in `good faith'* and for the person's `benefit.'*[62] The consent of the guardian or any person having lawful charge of a person under twelve years of age, or of unsound mind, subject to certain limitations of 'good faith' and the like, is considered as valid.[63] However, fear or misconception of fact invalidate an otherwise valid consent.[64]

Therefore, if a person having lawful charge, in good faith, for the benefit of the child under twelve years, without the child's consent, has the child operated for appendicitis by the surgeon knowing that the operation may cause death of the child but not intending death, then the person giving such consent as well as the operating surgeon are both protected by the provisions of this section even if death does occur.

In brief, the silver lining in the laws in case of mishaps resulting from acts to which a valid consent is given, is that, so long as an act is performed in good faith, for the benefit of the person who has given consent, express or implied, to suffer that harm or to take the risk of that harm, consent negatives the consequential criminal liability in case any harm does ensue provided there was complete absence of intention to cause death.

Therefore, where a surgeon operates on a patient knowing that it may cause his/her death, but not intending to cause it, and acting in good faith for the benefit of the patient, the surgeon commits no offence, provided that prior to the act, a valid consent was obtained. Consent, in such a case, would provide a complete defence in case of untoward consequences of any surgery provided all the negative ingredients which go against the validity of consent have been properly implemented.

---

[62]S.88, id.
[63]S.89, id.
[64]S.90, id.

The precautions hereinabove dealt with may be summed up as under:

- a person's consent to intentional causing of death is no consent under the law; it is because of this provision that mercy killing is still an offence;
- a person's consent to intentional causing of grievous hurt or to an act likely to cause death is no consent unless the risk is taken for his benefit. An over-riding requirement is that such a benefit should not be mere pecuniary benefit nor a benefit to be derived by any person other than the person harmed;
- a guardian may not consent to an act intended to cause death or which is an attempt to cause death except for the benefit of the minor and unless the harm caused is for the purpose of preventing death or grievous hurt, or curing any grievous disease or infirmity.

It has been a life long quest of the law-givers to visualise and provide for all possible eventualities. Accordingly, in a very restrictive provision, the law clothes the doctor with temporary guardianship in an emergency. Thus, where the patient is in no condition to give his consent, and or there is no other available person from whom a valid consent may be obtained, law cloaks the doctor, with temporary guardianship and enables him to take an independent decision regarding surgery, even in the absence of a consent provided he is acting in good faith and for the benefit of the patient. Here consent is totally dispensed with.[65] This legal provision enables a doctor to attend to emergency accident cases, street and midnight children and other exclusive cases who have no legal guardians but are in need of emergency services. For example, 'A' meets with a serious accident on the road and is immediately rushed to a hospital in an unconscious state. The

[65] S. 92, id.

surgeon is genuinely of the opinion that an immediate operation is essential to save his life and that any delay may prove fatal. In such emergencies, the doctor is not expected to wait till the patient recovers his senses, if he does recover at all. He operates without express consent. He would have committed no offence.

Applicability to Doctors

The concept of consent as applied to medical faculty, recognises the right of a patient to self-determination, imposing, for violations, a liability for damages under civil laws in tort and for punishment under criminal laws. One of the preliminary explanations of the importance of consent in medical practice and the application of its concept can be traced to the classic statement of an American judge, Mr. Justice Cardozo (1914):

> "Every human being of adult years and sound mind has a right to determine what should be done with his body, and a surgeon, who performs an operation without his patient's consent commits an assault for which he is liable in damages."[66]

It is consent which can exonerate a doctor from civil liability or criminal prosecution, acting as a guarding mechanism in case of accidental harm, but subject to all reasonable care and caution on the part of the medical man.

The right of an adult patient to be the final judge of whether or not to get operated for an ailment, after being informed of all the material facts which are necessary for him to know, to enable him take a deliberate decision, cannot be disputed and is based on the right to self-determination, awareness of facts and conscious assent. This right of selecting a course of treatment from the options available, presupposes the precise knowledge of the particulars on which the exercise of the choice depends and complete absence of feeling of constraint, so that nothing interferes in the exercise of free will of the patient.

---

[66] *Schloendorff v. Society of New York Hospital,* (1914) 211 N.Y. 125, N.Y. Ct of Apps.

However, in a doctor-patient relationship, the duty to disclose the factual condition versus the right to know, two options with vague colours and indeterminable shades, carries with itself the inevitable weighing of the gravity of the pros and cons in delicate scales. On the one hand, are the professional expertise of the doctor and the accompanying knowledge of the risk involved, and on the other, the anxiety of the patient and his near ones with regard to the prognosis and treatment which together create a chaotic condition and put a great deal of responsibility on the medical man. The law in such cases presumes existence of mutual trust in an otherwise 'fiduciary'* relationship.

In reality, whether the relationship between a doctor and a patient can be called `fiduciary' has not been touched upon in any statute. Whether the doctor is in a dominant position where he can take unfair advantage or whether the patient is mentally infirm or physically handicapped to such an extent that he could rebel against the rational decision of the doctor or yet whether the doctor has had to succumb to the wishes of the relatives in not disclosing the factual condition to the patient, has to be judged from the facts and circumstances of each individual case. No set rules exist and immense permutations and combinations of facts and figures would be needed to trace the factual position. In every case, the words of the Contract Act, 'unfair advantage' and 'undue influence' have to be adjudged with reference to the set of facts in differing contexts and no specific parameters can be enumerated to arrive at a conclusion, favourable or otherwise.

The doctor's dilemma does not end here. The medical attendant often finds himself battling between the legal necessity of keeping the patient informed of his medical condition and the knowledge that such disclosure would, in all probability, affect the patient adversely thereby enhancing the risk of a shock with its accompanying mental trauma which would, on the contrary, retard the chances of a good or even a reasonable prognosis. More often

*See Glossary.

than not, even the near relatives of the acutely suffering patient are hand in glove with the medical man, actually pleading with the doctor not to inform the patient about the impending peril to overcome his refusal to undergo the radical treatment so necessary to save the life. Such factors, intricately co-related with medical ethics, cloud the picture for the medical man who shoulders the responsibility of decisions involving human lives. For example, would it be appropriate to save the life of the mother by sacrificing the life of her unborn child or should he allow the mother to die so that the long prayed for precious progeny may survive? Should the doctor go on prolonging agony of the sufferer and the relatives merely in order to preserve life? Should he cut off a limb for saving the life against the wishes of the sufferer who does not want to lead a handicapped life merely because the relatives want the sufferer to live at all costs? These and many more situations cast a heavy burden on a conscientious doctor when he does want to do his best for the patient but law requires him to take steps which may affect the patient adversely.

Let us begin with the fact that the law requires every doctor to obtain a well-informed conscious consent from the patient in case of every surgical intervention except, for those not so rare cases, where the patient is not in a condition in which his consent can even be asked for and an emergency operation is required for his own benefit. Informed consent amounts to sanction of the patient to invade his body after being informed of all 'material facts' and a reasonable opportunity of satisfying himself of the procedures and the risks involved. The roots of informed consent lie in recognition of the right to self-determination and, in a way, submission to the feelings, intellect, individuality and values of the patient. Absence of such consent would legally and technically amount to an assault,* may be even an indecent assault, or use of criminal force,* or may be an unlawful invasion.

*See Glossary.

The question of informed consent is intrinsically connected with the doctor's duty to disclose the ailment to his patient, its extent, risks involved and probable prognosis. In fact, as the consent form establishes a privity of contract between the doctor and patient, it would be advisable to mention the names of any specialists intervening in the surgical procedures as well as the anaesthetist who is an important member of any surgical team. Problems can arise when the patient, genuinely or otherwise, feels and/or alleges that he was not informed of the inherent risks of the surgery or that the communication was not clear and material facts were not told to him and therefore he could not be said to have given an 'informed consent.'

For example, where the plaintiff, who had suffered from a neck deformity, became paralysed on the left side, from neck down, post-surgery and, although she had consented, she later alleged that the doctor had failed to provide her with all material information to help her to give a truly informed consent and that, had she been informed of the risk involved, she would have decided against operation, the Court rejected her argument on the basis that the doctor had provided material and sufficient information to enable the patient to decide whether to undergo operation.[67]

The vast expanse of medical science accompanied by different reactions and responses of every individual patient may make it impossible for a doctor to function if he is held liable for every possible adverse reaction. Nevertheless, the doctor must take reasonable care to explain all relevant and apparent details regarding the procedure and later rehabilitation, including an explanation of terminologies in a manner that the concerned patient understands. For example, merely stating that the treatment is conservative or non-conservative, invasive, non-invasive or less invasive, may not convey any meaning to the patient till he is made to understand

[67]*Hills v Potter and others*, (1983) 3 All ER 716.

their medical connotation and implications. The patient's allegation can be, firstly, that the operation was an assault on him since he had not given informed consent, the essential facts which could have made him take a contrary decision having been withheld from him and, secondly, that by failing to warn him of the inherent risks and other possible consequences, the doctor had been negligent.

The question which arises is: what would constitute material facts? In legalistics, such terms and phraseologies come to be judicially interpreted having regard to the circumstances of each individual case. For example, a risk of a minor disability may be an important fact, material in relation to a surgery for a minor ailment, but insignificant in case of a surgery essential to save the patient's life. Advancement in modern scientific innovations and progress in medical technology, like nuclear medicine, genetic engineering et al have enhanced the dimensions of 'facts' regarded as 'material.' Enormous practical variations and contradictions could arise leading to an eternal debate between the aggrieved and the medical man:

For example:

- Does duty to disclose material risks exclude the duty to disclose minor risks?
- What is the nature of the risk which can be labelled 'material'?
- Has material 'risk' to be weighed against the material 'benefit' of the specific treatment?
- Who would be competent to testify and guage whether the risk taken in a given case was essential and in the interest of the patient or not, in case a dispute on this point should reach a court of law? Non-medical members, however brilliant in their own field, sitting in judgment in a court of law and determing the propriety or otherwise of the decision of a medical man, is itself injudicious and the procedures in vogue have already installed inherent fears in the minds of the doctors who

have of late adopted over cautious tones in their practice much to the detriment of the sick humanity.

In a case[68] where a plaintiff was advised by a surgeon to have an operation on her spinal cord[69] to relieve persistent pain in her neck and shoulders and she was informed, prior to surgery, of the possibility of disturbing a nerve root and the consequences of doing so, but was not informed of the danger to the spinal cord, she sued the neurosurgeon, and the hospital governors claiming damages for personal injuries contending that the surgeon had failed to warn her of "all the possible risks inherent in the operation" and so she was not in a position to give an informed consent. Expert evidence* disclosed that there was approximately a 1% to 2% risk of damage to the nerve roots and a lesser risk of damage to the spinal cord.

Dismissing the appeal of the plaintiff, the judges stressed, in general, the duty of the doctor to disclose information as was reasonable, considering the circumstances of every individual case, which would enable the patient to take a rational decision, but, at the same time, said that it would be the doctor's prerogative to discuss remote risks of the procedures. The patient's age and mental state at the material time would be relevant to decide on this issue. Hence, what should be disclosed, for an informed consent, are material risks and a doctor cannot be held liable for non disclosure of remote risks.

To summarise, the law does require that patient should be explicitly informed of all material facts and the risk involved to enable him to take a conscious decision and the consent must be based upon the materials so disclosed.

---

*See Glossary.

[68]Sidaway v Bethlam Royal Hospital Governors and others, (1984) 1 All ER 1018.

[69]The operation consisted of a laminectomy of the fourth cervical vertebra and a facetectomy or foraminectomy of the disc space between the fourth and fifth cervical vertebrae.

Consent may be implied, for example, when it may not have been specified in words but is implied in the behaviour; or express, when it is clear, distinct and explicit in the language itself irrespective of whether it is recorded in writing or not. When a patient presents himself at the doctor's consulting room or out-patient's department, it is implied that he has consented to medical examination in the general sense. This normally implies a consent to procedures like inspection, palpation, percussion and auscultation. Oral consent, though valid, can create complications for the doctor in case of mishaps as, the onus will be on him to prove that consent had been given, though unrecorded. A duly witnessed oral consent would not suffer from this defect but then the credibility of the witness may yet be questioned. Thus a written consent should always be preferred as it has the advantage of being explicit and legally impeachable even in case of a legal dispute. For procedures involving withdrawal of blood for diagnostic purpose or a rectal or vaginal examination, oral consent, preferably in the presence of a third party who could be a witness if required, would do. For the more complicated procedures like endoscopy, arthroscopy and the like, written permission is preferred just as in surgical interventions. A consent form is an example of an agreement containing an express consent. These are subject to some limits, for example, the parties cannot agree to do that which would be regarded as contrary to public policy like illegal selling of human organs.

In order to help the patient to decide on a particular course, the doctor should deal with:

- diagnostics;
- dispensation of pharmaceutical drugs;
- monitoring the therapy towards cure/relief;
- referral subject matters;

- risk factors;
- bed rest/hospitalisation including economics;
- prognosis.

While on the subject of consent, negatively speaking, if a patient expressly refuses to consent, despite clear-cut, lucid explanations, then, technically, even if the patient passes away, the doctor cannot be charged for inaction. However, in reality, the situation is thorny and needs to be dealt with caution. In this very case, had the doctor decided not to operate, and the patient had died, the burden would have shifted on the doctor to prove that non-performance of surgery or non-administration of treatment was on account of refusal of patient to give consent thereto. In fact, legal opinion has gone to the extent that non-performance of an emergency operation and consequent death amount to negligence.[70] This decision could put the medical man in a crucial legal tangle to decide whether or not to operate and on which side of the court would the liability be less.

However, in such cases, the English courts have gone so far as to intervene and authorise procedures where the situation so required in order to save the life of the patient. For example, a thirty year old woman was admitted to the hospital with ruptured membranes and in spontaneous labour with her third preganancy but refused Cesarian section on religious grounds. The surgeon was clear in his approach that the operation was the only means of saving the patient's life and that the baby would not otherwise be born alive. In this case, despite express refusal of the patient, the court in exercise of its inherent jurisdiction considered the vital interest of the patient and the unborn child and authorised surgery.[71] In a somewhat similar case,[72] a thirty-four weeks pregnant woman

[70]See, *Dr T T Thomas v. Smt Elisa and others,* AIR 1987 Kerala 52-56.
[71]*Re S,* (1992) 4 All ER 671.
[72]*Re T,* (1992) 4 All ER 649.

who encountered injury in a car accident refused blood transfusion under influence of her mother who belonged to the religious sect, Jehovah's Witness, where the procedure is seen to be 'a sin and a bar to eternal salvation.' Despite her signing the form of refusal of consent to blood transfusion, following an emergency hearing, the judge authorised such procedure and the appeallate court later confirmed that if in a potentially life threatening situation, or one in which irrepairable damage to the patient's health can be anticipated, doctors or hospital authorities are faced with such situations of refusal for initial treatment and they have doubts as to the validity of such refusal, they should, in the interest of the patient and in the larger public interest, seek such a declaration from the courts as to lawfullness of the proposed treatment.

Also, the scope of consent cannot be enlarged at the discretion of the surgeon irrespective of the laudable motive. For example, consent to a Cesarian section, does not extend to the tying of fallopian tubes, even if subsequent pregnancy may have appeared hazardous.[73] Needless to say, in such a case, the court may easily have given a contrary verdict and held the doctor liable for having done exactly that which the patient had prohibited him to do. In one rare case,[74] the patient was to be operated for the removal of a diseased ovary. Before surgery, as a note of caution, the patient had told the doctor: "if you find both ovaries diseased, you must remove neither." During operation, the surgeon discovered that both the ovaries were diseased. Using his medical discretion, in good faith and as a step beneficial to the patient, he extracted both. He was sued on this account. However, the court held that having surrendered herself for operation, by implication, the patient had consented to removal of both the ovaries in case they were found diseased and therefore, the doctor had committed no offence.

---

[73]*Murray v McMurchy,* (1949) 1 All ER 497.

[74]*Beatty v Cullingworth,* (1896) BMJ 21st November, 1546 at 1548: See Mehta, *supra* n 1.

It is difficult to fathom what decision would have resulted from the Consumer Redressal Forum had such a case been placed before them. Could they have taken the broad protective decision in favour of the doctor who had so disregarded the specific instructions in this behalf, though in good faith and to save the life of the patient?

With regard to consent, hospitals and medical persons should bear in mind that:

- it should be an informed consent;
- technically, and strictly speaking, examination of a patient without his consent would amount to trespass, assault or even an indecent assault in some cases;
- it should be positive and not mere submission;
- in case of any doubt regarding the patient, it is better to obtain a written consent as a protection for the doctor;
- the consent form should clearly state that the doctor has informed the patient regarding the diagnosis, the procedure required, the alternative methods of treatment and his opinion on the resultant consequences in case surgery is not performed;
- consent should be free and not the result of fraud, undue pressure, duress, force, or fear;
- if it is obtained by misrepresentation or fraud, for example, by informing a patient that the operation is necessary to save his life or to preserve his health when in reality it was not required to save his life, it would amount to a fraud on the patient which would vitiate the consent;
- consent should not be accepted from one who is not eligible to give consent. For example, a minor or a person of unsound mind, even though they may sign a declaration, their consent will not be valid in law;
- in case of a child less than twelve years of age or a person of

unsound mind, a parent or guardian should give the consent;

- a consent may be invalid if it is unlawful. For example, an act like mercy killing which is prohibited by law;
- consent must not violate principles of 'immorality' and 'public policy.'
- for any procedures affecting matrimonial rights of a spouse like artificial insemination, sterilisation, hysterectomy, consent of both the spouses must be insisted upon.
- even where consent is given by the female patient to a male doctor for examination, it is better that a third female party or a female nurse should be kept in the room while examining the patient; it is a precaution worth taking;
- consent, being an agreement, two or more persons are required for its validity.

Conclusion

Consent has always played an important role in medical practice. However, a busy practitioner often disregards this mandatory requirement mainly because of the rarity of complaints and the pressures of medical life. Time is not far when distressing publicity, litigation and resultant damages, more particularly with the sweep of consumer activism, would bring in a realisation of the importance of these relatively simple procedures. As a pre-condition, regular forms are got signed and are insisted upon for all major diagnostic procedures or surgical operations in most of the hospitals in India. However, in the new order where 'accountability' holds a predominant placement, its importance cannot be overemphasised. With the wave of medico-legal litigations having existed in the West, spreading rapidly to India, increased frenzy of litigating against the medical man, with opening up of the newly introduced avenue of Consumer Courts, the parameters set out by Lord Denning[75]

---

[75]*Greaves & Co (Contractors) Ltd v Baynham Meikle & Partners*, (1975) 3 All ER 99, at 103-4 quoted *per* Nourse LJ in *Thake v Maurice*, (1986) 1 All ER 497, at 511.

should not be overlooked - that in carrying out an operation, the contract contains an implied warranty that the doctor would exercise "ordinary skill and care" of a competent surgeon, provided, no express guarantee, which no 'reasonable' medical man would advance, has been given to the patient. In today's times the value of written consent with reasonable clarity has increased tremendously. Remember the age-old adage: a stitch in time saves nine.

Medical Negligence

The sudden spurt in litigation against the professional man and an increasing equational gap in the doctor-patient relationship has opened up a Pandora's box for legal whips and brought to the fore, in a wave of what is being called 'awareness', of the always existing but rarely talked of 'accountability' of the doctor. The accusation of negligence, resulting in clinching liability on the medical man, howsoever stray a case, has made the doctor of today conscious of the onslaught of civil liabilities and criminal prosecution to which this community is vulnerable. It has made him extra cautious in his approach to the ailing human life invariably hanging by a fine thread which, God forbid, may snap at the very time he is being attended to by the doctor. The potential of 'malpractice suits', 'negligence liabilities', 'consumer complaints' and similar legal complexities have made the cautious doctor lose the earlier enthusiasm, nay anxiety, to attend to the sick and the diseased, howsoever complicated be the cases, as also the emergency ones, the time of the day or the risk to life and limb notwithstanding.

'Malpractice,' an adverse syndrome which has swayed the minds of human beings in recent times, literally means mala or bad and praxis or practitioner. In common medical parlance, it is used to refer to a bad or unskilled act by a physician resulting in harmful consequences to a patient. It could be either 'wilful' which would mean that "the physician or surgeon deliberately administers medicines or performs an operation which he knows and expects will result in damage to the health or in death of the individual under his care",[76] or 'negligent', which involves "those cases where there is no criminal or dishonest intent or object, but gross negligence of that attention which the situation of the patient requires".[77] Malpractice is thus the genus of which negligence is the species. Every act of negligence is a form of malpractice but the converse is not true as cases of professional misconduct may also be included in its ambit.

Historical Background

The first instance of an unscrupulous doctor being held liable for an adversely affected patient dates back to around 1727 BC, in the city of Babylon, where Hammurabi's Code was then in operation. This regulatory code prescribed the operating fees to be taken by the doctor as well as fixed penalties extending to cutting off the hand of the surgeon in case he inadvertently caused loss of an eye or the death of a patient in case of an operation resulting in an avoidable untoward consequence. Such and similar parameters developed the law of medical negligence and also gave rise to the concepts of 'due care', 'standard of care', 'good faith' and various other medico-legal notions.

Duty to Care *vis-a-vis* Negligence

The concept of 'care', inherent in the Hippocrates Oath,[78] gained momentum and steadily evolved into jurisprudential notions of 'due care,' 'duty to care,' 'standard of care,' 'reasonable care,' *et al.* From these developed the field of medical negligence, leading to doctor's liability under tort and crimes.[79] The breach of this duty

---

[76]*People v Lohman*, 2 Barb. (N.Y.) 216, quoted by George W Field, *Field's Medico-Legal Guide and Medical Jurisprudence 81* (1988) The University Book Agency, Allahabad.

[77]George W Field, *ibid.*

[78]*Supra* n 1.

[79]For details, see, Poornima Advani, "Duty to Care: From Hippocrates to Consumer Forums," paper presented at International Conference on Global Health Laws, New Delhi, 6-7 December 1997.

and/or taking the consequences complacently would entitle the person to whom harm has been caused, to accuse the person who was obliged to take care, as absence of mandatory requirement of care was treated as the preliminary seed of 'negligence.' It means:

"the omission to do something which a reasonable man, guided upon those considerations which ordinarily regulate the conduct of human affairs, would do, or doing something which a prudent and reasonable man would not do."[80]

To accuse a person of negligence, it is essential to establish a connection between the doer and the negligent act. The negligent act must be the causa causans (chief cause) of the consequent harm;[81] it is not enough for it to be *causa sine qua non* (similar cause).[82] For accusation to be effective, the rash or negligent act of the accused ought to be the direct, proximate and effective cause of the suffering inflicted or, may be, even the cause of death.

More specifically the parameters of medical negligence would require evaluation of facts and circumstances of the case:

- what is the standard of care required so as to amount to due care?
- who owes the duty to care?
- who owes the duty in case more than one person are involved in the act?
- to whom is the duty owed?

The scope of negligence is wide enough to cover liability in

---

[80] *Per* Lord Alderson in *Blyth v Birminghan Water Works Company*, (1856) 11 Ex 784: see Ratanlal and Dhirajlal, *Law of Crimes* 1196, vol 2, 23rd ed (1988) Bharat Law House.

[81] *In jure non remota causa sed proxima spectatur*: In law, the immediate, not the remote, cause of any event is regarded: Herbert Broom, *supra* n 46.

[82] Per Jenkins CJ in *Emperor v Onkar* (1902) 4 Bom LR 679, 682, See Ratanlal and Dhirajlal, *supra* n 80, at 1199.

tort as well as penalty in crime. In a civil claim, liability may be imposed even if there is no intention to harm but criminal responsibility is clamped only on the existence of a guilty intent (*mens rea*). The former requires proof only on a 'balance of probabilities' and would result in a claim for damages but the latter requires the matter to be proved 'beyond reasonable doubt' and would end in imposing a penalty, either fine or imprisonment. Attempting an over-simplification of the legalities, for the benefit of the medical man, the law of torts is primarily concerned with compensation whereas the criminal law is concerned basically with punishment and deterrence. As usual, the existence of negligence or the absence thereof leave a wide scope for judicial interpretation and is thus not easily assessable.

Criminal Liability

Under the Indian Penal Code 1860, section 304A prescribes punishment by way of imprisonment upto 2 years or fine or both in case of death caused by a rash or negligent act. However, neither 'negligence' nor 'rashness' are defined in the Penal Code.

Rashness and negligence, two common legal terminologies, do have very many similar ingredients. While rashness implies acting in the hope that no mischievous or adverse consequence would result, despite being aware of the likelihood of such consequence, negligence is acting without the awareness that a harmful or mischievous consequence will follow, but in circumstances which show that, had caution been exercised, the harm could have been avoided. Negligence is the genus of which rashness is the species. For example, a towel left inside the abdomen while conducting sterilisation, causing inflammation, necessitating repeat surgery and consequent death was clearly an act of negligence - the principle, res ipsa loquitir (things speak for themselves) being squarely applicable.[83]

[83] *Achutrao Haribhau Khodwa and others v State of Maharashtra,* (1996) 2 SCC 634.

Civil Liability

Tort duties could exist alongside contractual obligations. Tort liability may offer certain advantages to the plaintiff, for example, more generous rules for permitting recovery of damages, and potentially longer periods for commencing the proceedings subject to periods of limitation. A contractual obligation may provide an apparant advantage to the patient, for example, if a medical professional has guaranteed success. In *Thake v. Maurice,*[84] where the surgeon, after informing the patient that vasectomy resulted in irreversible sterility, without warning the couple of the risk that the effects could, at times, be naturally reversed, induced the husband to undergo the operation and a couple of years later, the patient's wife became pregnant, but ignored the signs being assured of the impossibility of conception post-surgery, the question arose whether there was a breach of warranty on the part of the operating surgeon. In the decision, the court declared that it was a breach of duty of the doctor and a failure on his part not to warn the patient of the slight possibility that he could become fertile again, post-surgery, which warning could have alerted the wife into seeking an abortion at an early stage. On this count, the plaintiffs were held entitled to damages. However, on the point of contractual obligation, the court looked upon the defendants contract with the plaintiff as one to "perform vasectomy" on the husband with "reasonable skill and care" rather than to sterlise him. Therefore, unless cent per cent success was guaranteed, bearing in mind that "medicine was not an exact science," with operative results being at times unpredictable, a doctor or surgeon could not be held liable for every eventuality which followed.

A somewhat similar matter arose in *Eyre v. Measday*[85] where, post-sterilisation, the plaintiff became pregnant and gave birth to a

[84](1986) 1 All ER 497.

[85]Eyre v Measday, (1986) 1 All E.R. 488.

child. An action was brought against the gynaecologist for damages, for breach of contract, contending that his representation that the operation was irreversible coupled with the failure to warn her of the minute risk that the procedure could, in rare cases, be unsuccessful amounted to breach of contract to render her sterile. Proceeding on the ground that the contract of the doctor with the patient was in respect of performing the surgery with skill and care but could not be extended to guaranteeing sterility, the court dismissed the appeal.

However, where a mother of three normal children had an abortion to terminate a fourth pregnancy and, at the same time, underwent sterilisation to prevent further pregnancies but again became pregnant, the Court concluded that the operation was performed negligently by the two doctors employed by the defendant health authority.[86]

Doctors Duties *vis-a-vis* Due Care

Technically, professional negligence in case of doctors would mean, "lack of reasonable care and skill... whereby the health or life of a patient is endangered."[87] Law does not imply a warranty that he (the professional man) will achieve the desired result, but only that he will use "reasonable care and skill."[88] In fact, courts have opined that when a person holds himself out as one who would give medical advice and treatment, he impliedly undertakes that he is possessed of skill and knowledge for the purpose.[89] A doctor is required, as part of his duty to care to his patient, to explain what he intended to do, and the implications involved, in the way in which a responsible doctor in similar circumstances would have done, and if there was a real risk of misfortune inherent in the

---

[86]*Emeh v Kensington and Chelsea and Westminster Area Health Authority,* (1984) 3 All ER 1044.
[87]*Supra* n 49, at 574.
[88]*Per* Lord Denning MR in *Greaves & Co (Contractors) Ltd, supra* n 75, at 103.
[89]*Dr Laxman Balkrishna Joshi v. Dr Trimbak Bapu Godbole,* AIR 1969 SC 128.

procedure, however well it was carried out, the doctor's duty was to warn of the risk of such misfortune.[90] The criteria, "whether he/ she is guilty of such failure as no doctor of ordinary skill acting with reasonable care could be guilty,"[91] has been highlighted, with relation to consumer disputes, more recently by the National Consumer Disputes Redressal Forum.

Prima facie, negligence is a legal and not a medical concept. Yet, definitions apart, a well demarcated distinction does exist between what a medical man is legally bound to do and what he ethically should do; one commands compulsion, the other projects an option. Agreed, the field of ethics spreads its wings more closely on the medical professional than on others; yet, moral duty and medical ethics cannot be viewed as legal compulsion.

However, despite absence of a binding legal constraint, his very profession casts a moral duty on the medical man to assist a patient with the expertise at his command. The doctor can refuse to treat anyone or respond to calls for home visits to unknown patients at odd hours. A private practitioner certainly has no such obligation.[92] However,the Apex Court has held a doctor under obligation to treat emergency accident cases,[93] while at the same time, and to the relief of the medical man, while recognising the risks involved in surgeries, has also observed that:

> " where the surgery is a race against time, the court will make greater allowance for mistakes on the part of the surgeon or his assistants, and give them the 'risk-benefit.'"[94]

Ethics apart, a doctor can refuse to treat a patient on the ground that he is unwell, or that he is preoccupied and therefore not in a position to accept responsibility of an additional case, or if

---

[90]*Chatterton v. Gerson and another,* (1981) 1 All ER 257.

[91]*Dr Sr. Louie and Anr v. Smt. Kannolil Pathumma and anr,* 1993 (1) CPR 422.

[92]For details, see *supra* n 10.

[93]*Pt. Parmanand Katara v. Union of India,* AIR 1989 SC 2039.

[94]*A.S.Mittal and anr v. State of U.P. and others,* (1989) 3 SCC 223, at 231.

the relation of the doctor with that particular patient are strained and the doctor fears that a genuine error in his judgment may be misinterpreted as a motivated misdemeanour, or if the patient reaches his consultation rooms without a pre-fixed appointment whereas there are other patients waiting with an appointment. Also, the doctor may justly refuse to treat a case where his professional specialised area does not coincide with the requirement of the patient. For example, if a patient comes to an orthopaedic surgeon to take his opinion on a dermatological problem, the former can reasonably refuse to take up the case.

The question arises, then, as to the exact point of time when the doctor's accountability initiates. For the lawyer, dealing with medical cases, this question bears a direct correlation to determine when, if at all, the doctor owed a duty to a particular sufferer. More apparently, the entire platform of accountability and liability gets set from the point of time when a physician accepts, or rather initiates, the treatment of a patient. From then on, he is bound to exercise due care and caution, utilising his professional knowledge and skill for the good of the patient. Here again, one may indulge on, which point of time can be referred to the moment of acceptance of the patient or the initiation of the treatment. Would it begin with the doctor embarking on the initial 'laying on of hands'? Again, the point of time when the doctor undertakes the care of a patient need not necessarily coincide with the time when the nursing staff or the hospital authorities undertake such care; these may all be dissociated in point of time and space. Normally, barring a few cases, where the margins can be cut and grooved, each case projects for itself the answers to these querries. Later, if the doctor desires to discontinue the treatment, he would be required to give reasonable time to the patient to procure another physician, perhaps even continue to treat him till he is safely placed under the care of another doctor.

Still, the subject matter is not all that simple. The complexities on the canvas run riot as more and more cases and possibilities are painted on it with a limitless variety of colours. The medical man's expertise, based on individual learning, qualifications, area of studies, professional judgment acquired through his personal experience and experiments on various patients over a period of time, is all too subjective. As the known rhetoric goes, no two doctors, both geniuses and experts in the same field, would agree on the same line of treatment and strategies, at the same point of time, creating confusion for the patient, who then turns to more doctors for their opinion getting more confounded than ever before. This factual position has been, in fact, accepted by the Courts:

"in the realm of diagnosis and treatment there is ample scope for genuine difference of opinion and one man clearly is not negligent merely because his conclusion differs from that of the other professional men..."[95]

Again, no two individuals with the same disease, respond to the same treatment, to the same extent or in the same manner. Therefore, it is well nigh impossible to quantify or qualify the degree of care, caution and skill that a practitioner is expected to exercise or has exercised or failed to exercise in the treatment of an individual patient. Legal high sounding debates have failed to lay down parametres for interpreting the term 'reasonable', and the phraseology 'reasonable skill', which again is explained to be "that which a prudent and reasonable man would exercise if placed in the same situation," all the terms being left to judicial interpretation based on the circumstances of each particular case. Unfortunately, like medical men, even judicial interpretation differs from judge to judge and time to time, creating chaotic confusion where nothing is certain. In the context of the doctor, the only measuring scale that can be prescribed is to say that the requirement is what would

---

[95]*Maynard v. West Midlands Regional Health Authority,* (1985) 1 All ER 635, at 638.

reasonably be expected of a practitioner of the same status, experience and qualifications, working under the same conditions. Thus in legal parlance, the level of expectation from the practitioner is set by 'peer review', or the application of the 'Bolam's test',[96] which would be the standard used to evaluate the reasonableness or the care, caution and skill of a doctor in a given case. The evaluation of reasonableness again, depends upon human ingenuity and can vary with circumstances and evaluating individuals.

In a case of accusation of medical negligence, once a doctor is found lacking in "reasonable skill or care," the onus is shifted on him to substantiate the correctness of the line of treatment adopted and the prudential methods followed or the diligence shown by him.

Over riding all the legalities, the permissiveness and the prohibitions, shines out the moral obligation which every doctor has got ingrained in him with the very selection of his career. As a human, and the one skilled to aid the human beings in general, he is morally bound to come to the aid of the suffering humanity, specially in case of emergencies and /or in circumstances requiring the use of his expertise.

In every case, the initial consultation, which marks the initiation of the doctor-patient equation, is the point of time when accountability begins. The journey may, in all probability, be a long one for once the faith is established, the relationship can last a lifetime. Much would depend on how the doctor initially projects himself : does he reflect the confidence that knowledge and

---

[96]Named after a negligence case Bolam v Friern Barnet HMC, (1957) 2 All ER 118 where the plaintiff had suffered fractures as a result of electro convulsive therapy; he complained that relaxant drugs had not been used. In fact, the use of relaxants was not encouraged by some practitioners due to significant side effects. The test states "(i) a doctor is not negligent, if he is acting in accordance with a practice accepted as proper by a responsible body of medical men, skilled in that particular art, merely because there is a body of such opinion that takes a contrary view."

experience impart to a person? Is he only after money? Would he be a good listener of his patient's woes? Is he one who would take a firm grip of a situation in an emergency coupled with clarity of communication? All these and a bundle of querries, though unspoken, go to form the preliminary impressions and decide the future bond of this introductory projection, which could go a long way to establish a well-knit doctor-patient relation.

Of course, the expertise in a particular field expected of a consultant specialising in that area, would be far greater than that expected from a general practitioner. Skill, training, experience in a particular speciality, reputation built up through the years, are all the hallmarks of a specialist for which he is preferred. The patient, placing his most precious possession in the hands of a particular doctor, whose specialised knowledge, skill and reputation alone would have induced him to seek out the doctor for his treatment, asserts his right to personal attention. This is all the more pronounced in India where faith and sentiments abide, where personalised care and treatment are greatly valued, the patient being primarily concerned with the specific doctor to whom he goes and none other.

Where a doctor does not possess appreciable skill in specific areas but has the qualifications to handle the case, even if he does attempt treatment, *albeit*, not successfully, he cannot be held liable on the ground that he should not have attempted the cure at all. The fact that he acted in good faith, for the benefit of the patient and that he had taken reasonable care and caution during the treatment, exonerate him from any blame even if the treatment failed to benefit the patient. The failure to benefit a patient alone does not make him liable for medical negligence. If a general practitioner indulges in surgery with adverse results, he could surely be accused of negligence and could be prosecuted.

Various stages in the doctor-patient relationship, each of them a potential firmament for an action on negligence, are :

- history taking,
- clinical examination,
- prescribing investigations which in the opinion of the doctor are essential,
- suggesting names of hospitals or doctors for investigations,
- diagnosis,
- guidance in the use of ancillary aids, if any, necessary for better and quicker prognosis,
- instructing the patient on dos and don'ts.

Due caution and restraint at every stage of his professional association with the patient are the prime pillars of 'accountability.' Suppose a heart patient has gone to a general practitioner in an acute condition in which hospitalisation is called for and, instead of directing the patient in consonance with his immediate requirement, the general practitioner merely gives him medication and allows him to go in the normal course, then if the patient dies, the doctor is surely at fault and could be held liable for medical negligence.

The conspicuous areas which could clamp liability on a doctor are:

- negligence by way of not recording proper history and complaints of the patient;
- failure to carry out essential investigations;
- wrong diagnosis;
- incorrect advice;
- negligence by way of not cautioning the patient with clarity on what activities the patient could undertake and what should be avoided;

- negligence in the management of the pre-operative procedure;
- negligence during surgery;
- negligence in the management of the post-operative follow-up;
- introducing untrained, inexperienced and unreliable staff in the team of the doctor's aides.

Recorded data has great veracity and value, unlike oral statements, and are accepted by courts as authentic documentary evidence establishing the credentials of the doctor unless proved otherwise. In the very nature of human behaviour, many communication gaps can occur, may be unintentional, by either the doctor omitting to convey or not stressing some significant instructions or the patient overlooking the instructions imparted, thus creating a dangerous gap. In such cases, factually, the patient may have been negligent in obeying instructions imparted by the doctor but if he just transfers the blame onto the doctor, a written chart can save the medical man many a litigation burn.

It is for these reasons that recording of a detailed medical history of the patient is of importance and emphasised during medical training but a point which many busy practitioners tend to overlook. Now with the spurt in medico-legal agitations, this complacency would have to be reversed, the non-existence of records would be far more detrimental and damaging to the busy doctor, in case he is sued, than an under-worked doctor who would easily be finding time to update his paperwork. Also, with the experience of the past and the well-reported incidents of the present, it can no longer be gainsaid that best of the over busy doctors, who have earned a name and reputation with years of hard labour and successful results in the fields of medicine and surgery, are not immune from litigation on charges of medical negligence.

On a more positive note, a proper history would also be of

great help to the doctor for diagnosis, treatment and prognosis, giving the doctor the much needed aid in evaluating the progress. It is therefore time for the busy doctor to wake up to a good organisation and method system for his day to day *clientele*, the faith and trust of the patients notwithstanding, which will prove to be rather a time saver bringing in its wake relief from the stress and strain of overwork.

The subsequent stages, the clinical examination and essential investigations undertaken in the interest of proper diagnosis and decision on the line of treatment to be adopted for good and speedy prognosis, are the basis of the doctor-patient relationship. Neither omitting the important investigations nor prescribing unnecessary ones for any other 'in-profession reasons' should be the principle. For example, failure to send a patient for x-ray when he complains of severe pain in his foot following fall of a heavy object on it, may lead to failure to detect a crack fracture of the long bones of the foot, a misery forever to the victim if the pain is allowed to become chronic. Therefore, omission of the minimum investigations, which harm the patient rather than save his money, does amount to negligence and needs to be guarded against.

As far as the investigative team is concerned, the radiologist, the sonologist or the pathologist, whosoever has handled the patient must even in an emergency, follow the oral report with a written one to the referring doctor who must, insist on a written report in order to retain complete transparency of records. Cases of diagnostic negligence are not unknown. The errors in diagnosis of the investigating team or a communication gap may, at times, lead to drastic decisions of the doctor causing irreparable harm to the patient. For example, where a pathologist diagnosed malignancy in a tumour when it was actually benign and the surgeon removed the organ without the least justification; or, conversely, if the pathologist wrongly reported on a malignant tumour to be benign, and the surgeon did not remove the organ leading later to spread of the secondaries and the demise of the patient, which could have been avoided, are clear cases of negligence. Failure to get the minimum required investigations does amount to negligence but acting on wrong reports of the analyst can land both, the doctor and the analyst, in a medico-legal net.

In a country like India, where poverty pervades the rural scenario and the urban areas are filled to the brim with slums, housing masses living below poverty line, rampant illiteracy, the patients are neither affording nor willing to undergo any investigatory procedures. The doctors have been upto now, by and large, relying on their clinical judgment for minor ailments or even at times for the most obvious diagnosis, yielding excellent results. On the other hand, in countries where money is plentiful, illiteracy rare and administration in capable hands, medical services are all under insurance cover and medical negligence litigation has been in the fore for over a couple of decades, the tempo of investigations is far more and absolutely mandatory.

Apropos the above-mentioned stages, that is, the history of the patient, the clinical examination and the results of the investigations, the doctor would, by now, based on his expertise and experience, have embarked on a firm diagnosis of the patient's malady, and he would then proceed with the ultimate aim of either attempting to cure his patient or at least relieve him of his suffering as much as possible depending on the ailment.

The subtle difference between a wrong diagnosis, which may be termed negligence, and a mere error of judgment has been recognised by the courts.[97] Diagnosis is based on subjective judgment of objective findings, interrelated with a number of factors, like the disclosure of essential facts, their interpretation and the clinical findings. Though factual correctness is surely expected from a medical expert specially where the investigatory findings point to

---

[97]*Dr. N.T. Subrahmanyam and anr v Dr. B. Krishna Rao and anr*, 1996 (2) CPR 247 (N.C).

a specific direction and no difference of opinion can lie, yet a doctor cannot be held up for mere inadvertance. In any case, much depends upon the evidence on record. In a singular case against a doctor where a complainant undergoing myelography and CT scan collapsed with paralytic attack, callousness and negligence alleged against the doctor were held, on evidence, not proved.[98]

However, the courts tend to give weightage to results of investigations *vis-a-vis* the course of treatment, for though not imperative, are yet an essential component of operative procedures. In a case where, ultrasonography, to determine the baby's position and size was not performed and the baby was born with Erb's palsy,[99] with Horner's syndrome,[100] a permanent disability caused by traction injury during delivery, the defence of the doctors that the head of the baby was spontaneously delivered but the patient did not cooperate with shoulder delivery, as a result of which, the baby was getting asphyxiated and was turning blue with a resultant danger to his life because of which the excessive force had to be used by the doctor, was not admitted nor was the excuse that the mother did not consent to a Cesarean accepted by the bench and a compensation of 1,75,000/- was clamped.[101] This appears to be a harsh decision against the doctor because every pregnancy does not go in for sonography and the doctor must have been between

---

[98] *Kuldip Singh Dhillon v Post Graduate Institute of Medical Education and Research*, 1996 (3) CPR 18 (CDRC, UT, Chandigarh).

[99] The Erb-Duchene type of palsy, commonly referred to as Erb's palsy, is evidenced by a combined lesion of the fifth and sixth cervical nerves, either below their junction or at Erb's point: See, Robert Duthie, George Bentley (ed)., *Mercer's Orthopaedic Surgery* 744, 8th ed (1983) University Park Press, Baltimore.

[100] Characterised by signs of paralysis of the cervical sympathetic (Horner's Syndrome): drooping of the upper lid, narrowing of the palpebral fissure, retrogression of the eyeball, contraction of the pupil, absence of sweating in the entire upper limb, the upper part of the chest, neck and half of the face, the area being accurately delimitied by the middle line: See, *id* at 745.

[101] Baby Ramya, represented by her father *K. Raji Reddy v Dr. Mrs. Aruna Reddy*, 1996 (1) CPR 244 (SCDRC, A. P., Hyderabad).

the devil and the deep sea seeing the condition of the baby. The case is surely one which could easily have gone in the doctor's favour but then, judicial wisdom does not follow a mathematical formula.

However, where a pathologist gave a blood group test report as 'A' positive, whereas two other hospitals testified the same as 'B' positive, the defence, that "some times fine clumping of red blood cells takes place leading to an error in conclusion," substantiated by authoritative books advising blood testing to be carried out in two laboratories before any blood transfusion to a patient, negatived the charges of negligence.[102]

Almost invariably, transparency between the doctor and the patient should be the hallmark at the time of the first consultation. The doctor ought to enlighten the patient whether surgery is imperative, or whether it could reasonably be avoided, resorting to conservative modes, for a while. In a vast number of cases, unless there is an emergency, or unless there was no option to surgical intervention, a knowledgable doctor would not rush the patient for surgery but would rather keep a watch on the patient under conservative treatment, even knowing that ultimately surgery may be the only answer. Generally, the doctor would, except in emergencies, give some breathing time to the patient for mentally accepting the surgeon's knife after satisfying the patient on all his querries and doubts. (See Chapter 2 for details on informed consent).

In any case, a medical man has to get over this crucially time consuming phase of collecting the patient's past data, his own clinical examination and the essential investigations, and simultaneously meet the challenge of over anxious and at times demanding patients and relatives, all of whom would be looking up to him for the diagnosis, line of treatment, prognosis, instructions regarding restrictions, if any, and the monetary involvement. Whereas the

[102] *Dharmendra Kumar Mishra v. Dr. Akhauri S. Sinha*, 1996 (2) CPR 192.

uneducated poor would look upto the doctor as their saviour, others, specially the partially knowledgable lot who know but little of the specialised fields, look forward to a clear-cut communication from the doctor. A few more methodic ones may even bring a written questionnaire to clear the cobwebs of their minds, for sickness and disease do lead to a chaotic condition, howsoever brave and peaceful the person is otherwise. Much would depend on the manner with which the doctor instills confidence in the patient and his near ones. Irrespective of whether the doctor is specifically asked or not, at this stage he is under an obligation to clarify every detail to the patient. If he has omitted to instruct a patient on important dos and don'ts and *per* chance some mishap occurs, to state that he was not asked for instructions on the point at issue would not be a valid defence.

Transparency with the patient and/or his relatives, if they do so intervene, is of utmost importance. The patient has a right to the doctor's frank opinion whether operation would bring a complete cure or only some improvement. It is also essential to enlighten the patient on his post-operative rehabilitative therapy, for nowadays, physical therapy, occupational therapy, speech therapy, etc. follow the operation and they are no doubt long term costly procedures. In fact, it is advisable to even inform the patient of the possible complications that accompany the procedure.

In most cases, a course of physical therapy is unavoidable and it is best to guide the patient to a proper centre, manned by a qualified physical therapist, not by an occupational therapist misrepresenting as the former, who would be the best to treat the patient for relief and rehabilitation and, in immobile cases, arrange for home treatment. The physiotherapist being qualified in this sphere must be left to decide on the line of treatment and select the appropriate modalities. Laser therapy or transcutaneous electrical nerve stimulation or yet a nebuliser for an acute respiratory problem all fall within the sphere of his expertise. Even apparently innocuous matters like manner of rest, change of mattress or the use of pillows or otherwise, the manner of getting up from the bed, instructions as regards dos and don'ts and the like, can make a significant difference to the patient's condition and comfort. Also, the physiotherapist ought to advise the patient on the appropriate manner and use of ancillary gadgets like sticks, belts, collars, walkers, crutches etc that would be required by the patient at every stage for better prognosis.

However, there will be cases where an occupational therapist would be the right choice for training the patient in 'activities of daily living' and developing intricate hand functions or in the general process of rehabilitation. Early and frank communication between the operating and rehabilitating doctors is essential for a good post-operative prognosis.

To sum up, every medical man ought to enlighten the patient with required guidelines in writing, duly signed by the doctor and, in view of the upsurge in medico-legal awareness and ongoing litigations, preferably countersigned by the patient. A copy can be kept in the doctor's records for future contingencies even though every patient need not be a litigant but the cautionary measure can save the doctor many a headache if brought before the recently introduced easy and inexpensive consumer redressal forums before whom quite a few doctors have been hauled up.

However, documentation of records to combat all ancillary accusations must be treated as a compulsory exercise for the doctor. If the records are transparent, the doctor has a valid defence against accusations of negligence. On the contrary, the doctor can have a grievance against the patient's negligence to abide by his instructions leading to his aggravated condition. A typical case would be of a patient taking a meal shortly before anaesthesia, despite being instructed otherwise in the written instructions handed over to the patient, or the case of a patient consuming larger doses of medication than prescribed and the like. All such litigations can be defended also on the principle of 'contributory negligence' of the patient. In such cases, while determining the quantum of damages, the court would deduct from the whole that proportion which is due to the patient's own negligence.

This theory of 'contributory negligence,' applicable in tort liability, is based on the principle that a responsibility accompanies a right. If the patient has a right to sue the doctor for inadequate medical treatment, there is a corresponding responsibility on the patient towards the medical man. This theory is also based on a well-known principle of English common law that contributory negligence bars the sufferer of harm from recovery of any damages even though the doctor may have been guilty of negligence to some degree.

More specifically, some of the defences available to the doctor are that the patient:

- has not revealed his history in its entirety and accurately;
- did not give an opportunity to examine the case properly;
- did not cooperate with the doctor for laboratory and other incidental investigatory tests like x-ray, cardiogram etc that were advised for proper diagnosis as a guide for future treatment;
- did not take his medication as prescribed;
- had inadvertantly or otherwise not disclosed related information necessary for proper diagnosis and treatment of the case;
- did not carry out all the instructions as regards rest, diet, etc;
- did not follow the other instructions of the doctor;
- failed to follow up his treatment as advised.

In a case where the patient suddenly moved his arm while the doctor was injecting him with a thin hypodermic needle causing it to break and the needle had to be removed surgically, the patient did not succeed in claiming damages from the doctor.[103]

In case of any surgery, the pre-operative, operative and post-operative regime should be adhered to scrupulously. Overlooking foreign bodies, incorrect dosage of injection, broken syringe needles, gangrene resulting from tight plaster casts, incompatible blood transfusions are some of the incidental mishaps to surgery which could be viewed as cases of negligence. So also where a doctor, looking after a patient, as part of a team, fails to inform another doctor of the patient's medical condition, as a result of which the patient suffers, would amount to negligence. A number of specialists, jointly participating in a surgery, thereby shouldering joint liability for inadvertence and negligence, is not new to the medical field and of crucial significance to the law of accountability. In case of a team of doctors, each member of the team will be deemed to have seperately undertaken the care of the patient when so assigned by a consultant; the latter, of course, would remain, as leader, responsible throughout the treatment and recovery because his undertaking of the care of the patient continues throughout the period of care. Failure to inject toxoid pre-operatively, a procedure followed the world over, or to administer antibiotics for 24 hours before surgery can result in civil or criminal liabilities in case of untoward consequences. However, in a given hospital, where a team of doctors are working, manning a particular unit, for example, the I.C.C. Unit, that by itself does not give cause to an aggrieved party to sue all the doctors of the unit. In other words, merely because doctors associate together as a team, the aggrieved cannot be compelled to implead other team members.[104] A direct connection between the negligent act and the particular doctor impeached are essential. During surgery it is essential for the surgeon to operate personally (and not leave it to his assistants as is reportedly

[103] *Supra* n 49, at 585.

[104] See, *M.L.Singhal v Dr. Pradeepathur and another,* AIR 1996 Delhi 261.

being done in hospitals), specially when the patient has engaged a specific doctor for the operation, and to have a duly qualified anaesthetist continuously monitoring the case, to assist him and, above all, to pay personal attention to the post-operative care. His responsibility does not cease with the operation but goes beyond into the patient's post-operative requirements. The practice of just remaining present during anaesthesia and then leaving the operation to others has put many a surgeon in the culprit's box and is a sure case of medical negligence. In addition, it would amount to a breach of contract between the patient and the surgeon unless, of course, consent for the surgery specifically includes the assistant and there is an understanding with the patient in this regard. Technically, the doctor cannot get away from his responsibility to operate personally even if the assistant is equally qualified and reputed unless a specific mention to that effect exists in the pre-operative papers.

Thus the surgeon would be well-advised to retain records of:

- physical examination of the patient;
- his remarks on the investigation reports;
- booking the operation theatre, the anaesthetist and the supporting staff etc;
- allergies, if any, of the patient which need to be guarded against;
- evaluation of the patient and any written instructions for the attending staff since the surgeon is not expected to attend to the patient all the time.

It is equally essential for the anaesthetist, even if he is only a visiting team member in the particular nursing home, to be fully equipped with all the drugs necessary, in case of an emergency, and not rely on the hospital authorities for the same. In case the patient suffers from any post-anaesthesia complications, the specialist would not succeed in transferring his responsibility on to the hospital on the ground that a particular drug required by him at the crucial moment was not available with them.

Equally significant is the post-operative follow up requiring the surgeon to take personal supervisory care of the patient during this phase. For example, if a patient complaining of tight bandage develops Volkman's Ischaemic Contracture,[105] the medico-legal invasion would certainly fall onto the doctor's scalp. Availability of the surgeon in the post-operative phase of surgery has been given great weightage by the judiciary in cases of allegations of post-operative negligence.

Issue of certificate

Caution is the key word for doctors, in a perpetual hurry, at times, sign blank letter heads for issue of certificates. In the current environmental set-up, they must necessarily be very careful to check every paper they sign, exercising caution before issuing certificates for any purpose, the contents being true to the best of their knowledge and belief. Verification of the authenticity of every statement, for example, unsoundness of mind or schizophrenia etc, incorporated in the certificate, if based on the statement made by others, is a must. Many have fallen victim to false certificates issued inadvertently by members of the medical community and, in some cases, are still languishing in mental hospitals where, every action of theirs and every sound that they raise is read as proof of madness and no one ever takes an inmate of a mental hospital seriously. It would indeed be medical negligence of the most inhumane type, even though indulged in without any malafide intention, to be an instrument in the conspiracy so as to confine a human being to the

[105]Volkman described a contracture in 1875 of the muscles of the wrist and fingers which followed tight bandaging of the arm in the treatment of fractures about the elbow. The tight bandage, he believed, was essentially due to ischaemia of the muscles, and that, as a result of deprivation of arterial blood, the muscles suffered from want of oxygen, the condition, he thought, was thus akin to rigor mortis: See, Robert Duthie, George Bentley (ed)., *supra* n 99, at 357.

dungeon undeservedly.

Conclusion

It is indeed impossible to enlist situations which can give rise to allegation of or an existence or otherwise of medical negligence. Even the adjudication of a given case is non-predictable and can differ from bench to bench of the same court and, may be, the mood of the judge too. Apparently, the age old respect for the medical profession has, rightly or wrongly, died its own death. In the earlier days it was a notion that a medical degree gives the person, however raw, a licence to kill. It is no longer so. Now the aggrieved patients do not accept such liberal rights for the doctor and do not hesitate to sue a doctor in case of mishap.

In the cut-throat competition amongst doctors, and the polluted environment with those in power, more often than not, routed in corruption and crime, no doubt some of the community members have indulged in unworthy practices but the penalty for this minority is being paid by even the best of the dedicated, honest and most skilled doctors. Today, the fair name of the entire fraternity stands tarnished for the offences of a few who have thrown moral values to the winds and have recklessly indulged in greedy, nay even criminal ventures.

However, considering that the environment all around, eight from the lowest to the top in the bureaucratic set-up, from the stray politician at the bottom of the ladder to the top brass, is smacking of scams, scandals and swindlers, to expect only the medical community to return its nobilitity without a smudge, is indeed expecting the impossible. If one may venture into the impossible terrain, most of the community is still dedicated, honest and caring. Yet the safeguards are essential specially for those who do not believe in the cut-throat systems and still wish to keep their heads above the polluted waters.

Planned Babies and Hired Mothers

The birth of Louise Brown in July, 1978, a professional career breakthrough for Dr Robert Edwards, the author of the invention, was no doubt an event for jubilation in the home of the newborn. A blessing to humankind, a triumph of science over nature, became too quickly polluted, revealing its dark side, opening up new avenues for trade - and where commerce makes its entry from the front door, litigation is oftentimes seen peeping through the back door. Courts have long since become the second side of the coin called 'money.'

Advancement of science and technology, in fields of embryo preservation, artificial insemination and *invitro* fertilisation (hereinafter referred to as IVF), lent a fresh hope to childless couples that they too can find the ultimate joy and happiness of parenthood so long denied to many. However, what started off as a laboratory innovation to bring light into the lives of deprived disheartened couples almost immediately misfired into the unethical anti-social game of commercialisation of reproductive organs. Economic dependence and misfired clamour in the name of women's rights have led to unmarried women voicing their "right to bear a child" and the "right to renting" of their reproductive organs, under the blessing of the advanced technologies, in the name of liberalisation of thoughts.

The scientists in their quest to alleviate suffering of humankind, including that of couples not being able to have progeny by normal means, have unwittingly opened up a Pandora's box of complex, debatable, legal issues involving moral and ethical complexities. This single scientific innovation now needs a body of mediating experts to resolve labyrinthine growth of issues that have cropped up between individuals as parents, real, hired or pseudo, the professionals who feel it their right to carry on their profession, whatever it be, responsibilities of all towards the 'miracle' child and his placement in society. This unintended, corrupt use of scientific research has in turn given rise to numerous legal issues of rare unfathomed nature. Today, prevention of gross misuse of science has become important in order to maintain a clean healthy society. The clearance of the cobwebs created by humankind is today the foremost heart-wrenching, brain-wrecking exercise for the law-makers, the law-dispensers and the intermediaries. Half-hearted measures and a few statutes to adorn the law libraries cannot sufficiently and effectively curb the mushroom growth. The unbridled misuse needs a sharpened legal sword and a solid legal shield to protect the age-old family unit that society has so meticulously carved out with ancient wisdom.

Hardly had the exuberance to this scientific achievement cooled down when 'baby sales' and 'womb hiring' struck a destructive note to the moral and social sanctity of the family fibre and delicate sublime infant-parent equation, giving rise to a society which would in time crumble under its own weight gathered by man's wanton entry into nature's domain and the society norms of matrimonial homes.

Varied complex situations have already been the subject matter of heated debates. Controversies raged, enmities and antagonisms multiplied and the adversely affected individuals have fumed and cried out in utter agony creating storms in medical, moral and psychological quarters. As of today, urgent legislation with coordinated effort of the doctor, lawyer, social scientist, legislator and the machinery enabling rigorous implementation of norms so arrived at, is required to effectively tackle the problem, curb the commercial misuse and to determine a workable solution.

ARTIFICIAL INSEMINATION

Historical background

Multiple theories to correlate processes of artificial insemination to similar practices prevalent in ancient eras, aiming at preservation of genetic lineage of the family, aiding the childless to conceive, have oft been attempted. Some similiarities are claimed to have been traced. As an example, historians have cited the practice of *niyoga*, prevalent amongst Hindus by which a kinsman was appointed, in a spirit of *dharma*,[106] to beget an issue by a widow or wife of an infertile husband with this 'modern' technology.[107] In such cases, after child birth, the kinsman and woman held each other in respect, their relationship being looked upon as that of father-in-law and daughter-in-law. Such a woman was called *Kshetra*, meaning a field, and the child *Kshetraja*, meaning born out of the field.

However, on the scientific front more recently, with profound ingenuity, it was Schenk who, in 1880, struck upon the idea of experimenting with fertilisation of oocytes of mammalian rabbits and guinea pigs *invitro*. However, for quite some time no positive results were obtained apparently due to failure to use an effective medium for fertilisation of the eggs. Experiments continued relentlessly till one fine morning the virgin seed of what was to develop as an expansive field of genetic engineering sprouted in

---

[106]*Dharma,* as derived from the root *dhru,* means "to uphold, to support, to nourish", used to indicate primary duties and responsibilities. See P V Kane, History of *Dharmasastra (Ancient and Medieval Religious and Civil Laws in India)* 1, vol 1 (1968) Bhandarkar Oriental Research Institute, Poona.

[107]See, Paras Diwan, "Technological *Niyoga* and *Nirodh* and Social Engineering Through Law" 22 *J.I.L.I.* 445, 449-50 (1980).

the fertile soil. It had taken exactly a century for the historic day, which was to bring success to science itself, to dawn. The two doctors, Patrick Steptoe and Dr Robert Edwards,[108] having successfully resolved the problems encountered by the earlier research workers, had performed a Herculean feat, marking a victory of science and the scientists in the world of 'genetic engineering.' On 28 July, 1978, Louise Brown was born in Great Britian as the first *invitro* baby.[109] The baby marked man's victory over nature.

For a couple of decades, rigorous experiments to improve artificial fertilisation techniques were systematically conducted. Later, developments in the methods of cryopreservation of embryos, artificial insemination and surrogate motherhood enabled scientists to light the lamp of hope in a number of disheartened childless couples. However, even before the cinders of celebration accompanying the 'divine' discovery could burn out, the 'criminal' misuse of the procedures through commercialisation, opening up a new market in the field of reproduction, had already been invented. Getting babies manufactured to specification, without having to bear the pains and responsibilities of pre and post-natal care, became a possibility. A new market ensued. Genetic seeds for sale and wombs on hire became commercial commodities. Specialised agencies to provide wombs on hire from economically poor and needy sections of society helped to regulate an upcoming market. A virgin seed had sprouted into wild growth.

Many unimagined situations arose which necessitated immediate legal intervention. For example, the rights regarding disposal of surplus human embryos, which in reality were capable

---

[108]Reminiscing over those times, says Edward "... with Patrick Steptoe, began the lonely and frustrating pathway that ultimately led to the joy of the birth of Louise Brown. There were no funds freely available, nor any encouragement to begin or continue the work, while a chorus of criticism accompanied every advance in our attempts to introduce the methods." See R G Edwards and Jean M Purdy (ed), "Preface" *Human Conception In Vitro,* vii (1982) Academic Press Inc.
[109]*Ibid.*

of being developed into babies, single women desirous of parenting by-passing the need of having a male partner; and on the other hand, married normal women wanting to hire other's wombs thus throwing to the winds the norms of morality, nature and principles of society formation, were some of the issues that faced the developed countries like a thunderbolt.

Embryo cryopreservation

Accumulation of a large number of frozen oocytes and embryos, resulting from multifollicular stimulation required routine destruction of the 'excess' embryos which gave rise to the need to develop a method of preservation. Need for man has always been the mother of invention and this particular need culminated in innovating procedures for embryo cryopreservation. Today, the process has been so perfected that embryos can be preserved and nurtured into babies at will.

The first successful pregnancy from impregnation of cryopreserved and thawed embryo dates back to 1983 when Trounsen and colleagues successfully brought into the world Zoe Layland on 28 March 1984 at the Queen Victoria Medical Centre, Melbourne.[110] About six months later, on 17 August 1984, the world's second baby, resulting from IVF with a preserved embryo, was born to Ms Margaret Brooks, aged 33 at the same Australian hospital.[111] The well developed baby weighed 8.16 lbs and was named John after Professor John Leftend who performed the historic fertilisation. The success of pregnancy, not only *invitro* with fresh gametes but also with preserved ones, was established beyond doubt. Today, virtually at any stage of development of the embryo, from zygote to blastocyte, freezing can be successfully achieved and integrated with the procedure of IVF.

---

[110]See, Joseph Bellina and Josleen Wilson, The Fertility Handbook: A Positive and Practical Guide (1986) Penguin Books.
[111]Ibid.

The successful preservation procedures have proved to be a boon to many couples locked in serious compulsions. For example, the freezing of gametes prior to exposure to radiotherapy, to be utilised at a later date, has led to some succour to unfortunate couples keen on their rare ancestral genes in the child but who would otherwise run the risk and potential danger of giving birth to defective babies through conception post-radiotherapy.

However, with human ingenuity being what it is, a number of legal and ethical issues of an increasingly humane and personalised nature, affecting individuals and society at large, have cropped up. The preserved gametes have acquired the colouring of 'property', perhaps 'moveable property' would be the more accurate term, thus undoubtedly becoming objects with 'ownership' and/or 'possessory' rights. Furthermore, after much hair-splitting on the point of preservation *versus* destruction, the gametes have been adjudged as future 'beings' and the issues of 'right to life' guaranteed by laws have also cropped up.

The primary issue of right of ownership *versus* possession and the consequential control over the fate of the embryo have ensued into sharp legal battles. In cases where embryos are preserved for long, change in circumstances due to ever new situations have complicated matters further. For example, the owners (being the parents of the future baby) may have parted ways and may no longer be interested in joint ownership thus leading to greater scope for individual disputes.

Astounding innovations in genetic engineering have swept the world, but unfortunately developed a gene market resulting in high stake commercialisation. Various situations can be highlighted. For example, a couple undergoing infertility treatment may, during the process, want to abandon the idea of having their baby and may find it advantageous to dispose off their embryos by sale. In another situation, a couple may desire to sell off the excess embryos or even preserve embryos only in order to sell them for material gains. Friendly aid to infertile couples is one of the possibilities. Apparently, the field of bio-genetics carries with it an immense potential of leading to commercialisation thus stimulating problematic issues. Needless to say, legal intervention and clarity with appropriate regulatory legislation, imposing a ban on commercialisation on the ground of violation of societal norms and public policies are essential if we are to maintain the basic family structure.

Indications

Artificial insemination has been broadly classified into three categories: AIH (Artificial Insemination Homologous), wherein the husband's sperm is used;[112] AID (Artificial Insemination Donor), where the sperm used is of a donor;[113] AIC (Artificial Insemination Combination) wherein the husband's and the donor's sperms are comingled.

By and large, artificial insemination of the first type is preferred as it does not pose any legal issues of significance. However, the second and third processes are potential potholes of disputes and hot spots needing legal intervention. The Roman Catholic Church and Orthodox Judaism both forbid its use, though in the latter case the offspring is seen as legitimate, while under Roman Catholicism, the offspring is treated as illegitimate and the act itself as adultery.[114] The thought processes of the religions of the Orient were somewhat similar.

Analysis

In his textbook of *Medical Jurisprudence and Toxicology*,[115] Modi

---

[112]Robert Franklin and Dorothy Brockman, *In Pursuit of Fertility* 186 (1991) Henry Holt and Co, New York.

[113]*Id* at 234.

[114]*Supra* n 9, at 151.

[115]C.A.Franklin (ed) 349, 21st ed (1988) N.M.Tripathi Publication, Mumbai.

describes the indications for artificial insemination:

"incurable defects in the husband's semen rendering him incapable of procreation; mental disease in the husband; hereditary disease in the husband of such a kind as to contraindicate paternity; and Rhesus incompatibility resulting in failure of children to survive because of erythroblastosis and the husband is homozygous Rhesus positive."

Legal issues

With induction of artificial insemination as a way of reproduction, various legal issues have arisen:

- whether AIH amounts to consummation of marriage?
- should prior consent of the husband be made mandatory for a married woman with a living husband in case of AID?
- is it a basic human right of a woman to have a child even by AID?
- if so, then, does the child have any rights of entry into the family tree of the husband?
- whether resorting to AID, without informing or without the consent of a woman's husband, should be prescribed as a 'fraud' in marriage?
- whether AID without the consent of the husband should be made a specific ground for divorce on the ground of adultery or otherwise?
- whether AID amounts to adultery on the part of the wife?
- should the penal laws be made applicable in case of violation of these norms?
- what would be the status of the child born of AID in terms of legitimacy?
- if the husband of such a woman is not willing to accept such a

child, does the mother have any right to use the name and / or surname of her husband for the child?

- in such cases, is the donor under a legal obligation to provide his name to the child?
- what would be the custodial and visitational rights of the donor who is the genetic father?
- would the rule of prohibited degrees be operative to a child of AID? Could the child be said to be within the prohibited degrees of relationship with the relatives of the husband of the woman whose child he is or with the genetic father? This clarity is essential as the personal laws of some castes and communities in India prohibit marriage within prohibited degrees of relationships;
- what would be the rights of inheritance of a child born of AID *vis-a-vis* a consenting and also non-consenting husband?
- what norms, rules and regulations should be made for the attending physician who performs AID?
- what are the responsibilities and liabilities of the donor, the mother and / or the doctor in case a defective child is born with AID?

These and many more questions affecting human relations, family units and societal norms, do arise and need an answer from legal experts and law makers, without further complacency, as the cases are multiplying by leaps and bounds and without clarity, soon the courts would be filled with endless litigation with no available guidelines.

In the United Kingdom, a Departmental Committee, studied the problem from a broad perspective and advised that:[116]

[116] *Supra* n 10, at 269.

- the practice of AID should be strongly discouraged but should not be regulated by law, or held to be a criminal offence;
- the birth of a child as a result of AID, to which the parties of the marriage consented, should be a bar to proceedings for nullity of marriage on the grounds of impotence;
- there should be no alteration in the procedure for registration of birth or of the laws relating to legitimacy;
- insemination of a wife with donor semen without the consent of the husband should be made an additional ground for divorce or judicial seperation and provision made distilling her alimony either under the Civil or the Vagrancies Acts.

On the domestic front, in the Indian sub-continent, with the flora and fauna of religions and cultures added onto the indigenous people, its multifarious castes and communities, their varied customs and norms, non-implementation of Constitutional requirement of a Uniform Civil Code applicable to all citizens, with conflicting personal laws being different even amongst the members of the same religion, differing ethical, moral and religious concepts amongst crores of illiterate, uneducated, poverty ridden masses, with uneducated politicians and contradictory policies inducted much too often at the helm of affairs for running the nation, with the intelligentia having become mere passive observers of the constant regression in the nation's development, satisfied with doing their bit by their muffled voices published in media, the effects of induction of AID as a way of reproduction in society would be, to say the least, quite mind-boggling, revolting and unmanageable.

Further analyses of the legal issues follows:

Artificial Insemination and Adultery

Whether introduction of a 'spurious' child by AID into the family of the husband amounts to adultery has formed the subject matter of legal debates. Also, whether imposition of such a child in a matrimonial institution, without the consent or knowledge of the husband, should be considered as a crime in marrige or whether it should merely form a civil ground for divorce, are controversial issues have been discussed at seminars the world over.

This issue was formally brought up for the first time before a Canadian Court in *Oxford v Oxford*[117] where the wife gave birth to a child undisputedly outside the marriage norms, for while she was in England, her husband had all along resided in Canada. The charge of adultery brought in by the husband was sought to be defended on the premise that she had conceived the child by artificial insemination under medical care. The court while rejecting her defence stated:

"....that no authority can be found declaring, directly or indirectly, that 'artificial insemination' would constitute adultery is not to be wondered at. This is probably the first time in history that such a suggestion has been put forward in a court of justice."[118] They concluded:

"Any act on the part of the wife which does that (referring to AID) would, therefore, be adulterous. That such a thing could be accomplished in any other than the natural manner probably never entered the heads of those who considered the question before."[119]

Technically speaking, it would appear that due to the inherent and wide differentiation in their objectives and procedures, AID and adultery will have to be viewed independently and evaluated threadbare, keeping in mind the human needs and emotions, the nation's religious and cultural values, and above all, the well formed society norms. The differences are obvious. Whereas adultery is invariably an emotional and secret affair and can remain hidden for life, AID is a result oriented voluntarily sought procedure resorted

---

[117](1921) 49 Ontario Law Report 22.
[118]Id at 257.
[119]Id at 258.

to after conscious decision. Whereas the objective of AID is invariably to have an offspring, adultery rarely has parenthood as its chief objective.

Presuming for the sake of argument that AID would amount to adultery, some intellectual exercise would still be required to resolve its implications. It is by now common knowledge that sperms are a preservable commodity and, if well processed, can last for a considerable length of time. As a natural corollary, they can be used even after death of the donor giving rise to the question that if, in a given case, sperms of a dead man are used to impregnate a woman, would she have allegedly committed adultery with a dead man? Can the medical man, who performs insemination, be held guilty of aiding or abetting adultery?

While one cannot undermine the utility of this scientific invention, ill effects of AID utilised by a married woman without her husband's consent need not also be underrated for it is a certain assault which must uproot the very essence of a marital relation by introducing an element foreign to the family of the husband, surreptitiously destroying mutual faith and trust which are the essentials of a marriage and are inborn in matrimony. Also, since the entire aim of AID is birth of a child, issues such as inheritance rights of the child and the question of its legitimacy need utmost clarity.

Appropriate legislation to deal with all such interrelated problems, more specifically how the divorce laws and/or matrimonial crimes should deal with the varied situations, is surely the call of the hour. However, even before any legislation is carried out, following issues need a definite answer:

- whether AID should or need not be classified as adultery;
- whether AID without the consent of the spouse should be dealt with only as a specific ground for termination of marriage;

- whether the unlimited scope of mental cruelty would cover the procedure undergone by the wife and a specific mention be made merely to avoid any doubts and debates.

Artificial Insemination and Consummation of Marriage

The personal laws as they stand today, with regard to consummation of marriage, are as follows:

- section 32 (a) of the Parsi Marriage and Divorce Act, 1988, treats non-consummation of marriage owing to wilful refusal of the spouse within one year of marriage as a ground for divorce;
- section 25 (i) of the Special Marriage Act, 1954, gives a right to both the parties to annulment of marriage;
- section 12 (1) (a) of the The Hindu Marriage Act, 1955, prescribes remedy of annulment of marriage to the wife only, on the ground of non-consummation owing to impotence of the husband;
- section 2 (vii) of the Dissolution of Muslim Marriage Act, 1939 enables a woman, married under that Act, to obtain divorce on the ground that she, having been given in marriage by her father or other guardian before she attained the age of 15 years, repudiated it before attaining the age of 18 years with an added proviso that her marriage has not been consummated.

None of the statutes deal specifically with the legal position in case a married woman resorts to AID without the consent of her husband, when her marriage itself has not been consummated. A peculiar situation would arise when a husband is physically impotent and such fact is withheld from the wife at the time of marriage. Having committed a fraud on her already, should he also have the right to deprive her of motherhood which she desires to fulfil by artificial means through AID? In the alternative, would the position be different if there is no fraud committed in the case of a relatively impotent husband? Such and many other questions need to be answered before passing legislation thus sealing the fate of those women who may want to resort to AID even without the husband's consent under compulsive circumstances.

In *R E L v E L*,[120] the wife of a psychologically impotent husband who was unable to consummate marriage decided to get herself artificially inseminated by her husband's seed. However, she went through the procedure for about twelve months without perceiving any results. Being fed up with her forlorn situation, in utter ignorance that she was already impregnated, she decided to leave her husband. Subsequently, a child was born. The woman however was determined not to return to her husband. She moved the court for a decree of nullity of her marriage on the ground of non-consummation.

The court was faced with a peculiar situation. Factually, the marriage was not consummated but a child, genetically belonging to the mother and an estranged father, was born during wedlock. Despite the existence of a child, the court negatived an implication of consummation of marriage to be drawn merely by the wife getting herself artificially inseminated with her husband's seed. The court declared such marriage as null and void although the decree did have an effect of stamping illegitimacy on the innocent child. Yet artificial insemination homologous was unequivocally demarcated from consummation of marriage.

Artificial Insemination and the Unmarried Woman

With a general clamour for women's rights renting the air, more liberal views on unmarried woman's rights have hit the cosmos. Question is: if a woman decides against a male partner in her life but wants to fulfil her desire of motherhood, what would be her and the child's placement in society?

One case on this subject reported from the State of New

[120] (1949) *Probate Division* 211.

Jersey[121] involved an unmarried woman, with an intense desire of motherhood, who came to an understanding with her boyfriend after being with him for two years, to get him to be the donor wherewith she could resort to insemination. Not being able to summon cooperation with any physician, the duo familiarised themselves with the procedure and attempted it on a number of occasions spanning several months when the boy used to frequently visit the residence of the girl. Ultimately, she succeeded in achieving conception but, some time in the third month of her pregnancy, the two year old relationship came to an end. A child was born. The father, still an unmarried young man, filed a suit stating that since he was the genetic father and was desirous to fulfil his role, he should be given visitation rights of the child. The situation turned challenging and both sides took up their cudgels to litigate.

The question for decision before the New Jersey Superior Court was whether an unmarried man could be considered to be the natural father of a child and given visitation rights or should he be denied this right because the lady had conceived through AID. The court, while refusing to clarify the propriety of unmarried persons resorting to artificial insemination, recognised public policy considerations, that it is in the "child's best interest to have two parents"[122] and while allowing the petition, the father was given an additional responsibility for support and maintenance of the child.

This is only one case, but, considering the complexities of the subject matter, various situations can arise. The woman can get herself inseminated by an unknown donor's seed, in which case, if the genes are bad, she might have a hard time indeed.[123] In case

---

[121] C M *v* C C, 152 N J super 160, 377A 821, 2 ed (1977), See Mr George P. Smith, "Sexual Autonomy or Government Intervention : Artificial Fathers and Surrogate Mothers" paper presented at World Congress on Law and Medicine, Indian Law Institute (New Delhi, 1985).

[122] *Ibid.*

[123] Poornima Advani, *Causes of Antisocial Behaviour and Crime - A Socio & Medico-Legal Perspective* 7 (1990) Gopushi Publishers, Mumbai.

she goes in for a known donor, he, as the genetic father, may claim visitation rights and her entire purpose of evading the responsibility of a male partner may be reduced to naught. In the third alternative, she may, perhaps, get the donor as well as a surrogate to create the child with the clear intention of adoption, having to rely on the State laws governing adoption to determine whether, as a single woman, she is eligible to adopt.

These situations, although piquant, do need a clear-cut legal direction. Probably, law can come to her aid, allow her to adopt a child as a single parent, with no visitation rights to the genetic father. But then, the other side of this coin is that these steps might work towards rupturing the institution of matrimony and establishing new society norms. How would society accept such mothers and their off springs?

Perhaps a socio-ethical dialogue is needed to lay open the thought processes to such problems.

Surrogate Motherhood

Often referred to as 'parenthood by proxy' or 'renting of wombs' in consonance with its commercial ingredient, the goods, that is, the child being an outcome of *invitro* fertilisation, involves the appointment or hiring of a compatible woman to bear the child for the whole or part of the gestational period as the circumstances might require. The 'surrogate mother', inseminated with the sperm from the husband of an infertile woman, or the oocyte of a normal woman who cannot bear the child due to physical incapacity or even one who wishes to by-pass the painful process of child bearing and delivering the child, would carry the foetus full term and after delivery hand over the offspring to the hiring client.

The first surrogate mother to have given birth to a baby against money was on 4 January 1985 in Britain. The surrogate, Kim Cotton, a 28 year old married woman with two children of her own had been paid 7,475 dollars to bear the baby after having been inseminated with the hiring husband's sperm for probably an American childless couple.[124] Within hours of birth, the Social Service Director, Alan Gorst, the Council authority in North London borough of Barnet, claimed the child on the grounds that the Council was responsible for the welfare of all babies born in the area and opined that any money transaction involving a child would be unlawful.[125] In the words of Kim, "thanks to Social Services, the baby, she had two mums, neither of whom could take her. The press christened her 'Little Miss Lonely' while her parents fought a High Court battle to claim her." Finally, Baby Cotton, as she came to be known, and her rightful parents, flew secretly out of the country, to start a new life abroad, as a family.[126]

Today, it is not uncommon for a couple to grow the fertilised egg from their respective ovum and sperm to full maturity of nine months and have their baby born from another woman. However, the natural mother, who has carried the child for nine months, nurtured the baby *invitro*, suffered the pangs of pregnancy, to whom nature had joined the baby by the umbilical cord, is not the genetic mother!

Initially meant for the forlorn childless married couples, the procedure has in time gained popularity even amongst men and women who wish to have children by-passing the institution of marriage or where either spouse is unable to fulfil his/her or the other's basic instinct of parenthood thereby creating a class of single parents who hire surrogates to bear the child for them and then adopt the child, knowing that the child is at least fifty per cent their own, with their ancestral genes at least in part. Many prospective parents get more satisfaction through such children as in regular adoption the child is a complete outsider to the family tree.

---

[124]See Kim Cotton, *Second Time Around* 5 (1992) Kim Cotton, New Barnet, Herts.

[125]*The Hindustan Times* (New Delhi ed) 6 January 1985.

[126]See Appendix D-Personal message from Kim Cotton to surrogates in a letter addressed to the authoress.

The methodology is also gaining momentum amongst affluent married women who can bear their own child biologically but prefer to purchase the luxury of being saved the normal pains and inconveniences and still have their own progeny. This hiring of another woman has many attractions for the affluent as they do not have to 'waste' nine months and odd in carrying a child and can maintain their trim figure intact and socialise all the time. This process also appears to be gaining popularity amongst the career conscious entrepreneurs and professionals who have no motivation for suffering the pangs of pregnancy and labour or rather, on balancing priorities, do not find it worthwhile to 'waste' precious time and energy for attaining the status of motherhood when there are others who can be paid to do the needful for them while they continue in their careers.

The introduction of surrogacy in motherhood has proved to be extremely piquant. A procedure meant to provide the missing ingredient and yield succour to a female partner, unable to carry a foetus to full term, has been misused, illused and commercialised, raising queer issues regarding the rights of the third party involved in the process. Its usage by the single woman who wants to give a side walk to the institution of marriage and at the same time have a child, with another woman bearing the child, who would belong at least fifty per cent to her genetically; its misuse by the affluent who desire to have their genetic child coupled with the luxury of the wife not having to bear the pains of procreation, have popularised the procedure more than it was intended for. Is it any wonder that commercialisation should have swept into surrogacy, an otherwise innocent mode of aiding those barred from enjoying motherhood by physical handicaps?

Many feminists have commented that the term 'surrogate' for the carrying or gestational mother is inappropriate: if anyone is a surrogate mother, it is the 'social' mother.[127] These transactions, often finalised by the commercial surrogacy agencies who engage lawyers to draw up the agreement, are now entered into between the carrying mother and genetic parents, through written contracts which specify rights and duties of the parties concerned including one or more eventualities and also compensation to be paid to the surrogate.

In some countries, commercialisation has taken such roots that even classified advertisements calling for applications from willing women appear in popular newspapers.

"Infertile couples looking for a woman to bear a child. Child would be adopted by the couple at delivery. Compensation and all expenses paid. Correspondence strictly confidential. Respond to..."

run the ads. Even in India, such advertisements have appeared in the media. Reads one ad:

"Wanted motherhood on loan. For a happy, educated and childless couple, a woman who can bear a child. Required for the purpose, those seperated or unmarried but adult, may please contact. Married woman should have the consent of the husband. Adequate compensation. Baroda woman first preference."[128]

Another ad reads:

"Wanted surrogate mother to bear child for a young, rich, good looking Brahmin couple. Very large compensation. If required comfortable and secure future life assured..."[129]

Significantly, the advertisements do not express any bar to religion or caste of the carrying mother which some of the conservative communities may find objectionable.

---

[127]See, Regina Graycar & Jenny Morgan, *The Hidden Gender of Law* 232 (1990) The Federation Press.

[128]*The Pioneer* (Delhi ed) 19 April 1995.

[129]*The Pioneer* (Delhi ed) 5 August 1994.

Suffice it to say, that with commercialisation of this process, the womb of the seller mother has become a biological incubator to be hired out on payment of money converting her from a feeling and emotional human mother to a machine manufacturing goods. In its finer analysis, the process is nothing but sale of an unborn human child, a child which would be formed and nurtured by nature as an inseparable part of the surrogate mother who will carry it to full term, "till birth do us part." Having received an embryo, she has to surrender her entire instinct of motherly love - the most sublime and divine of emotions that human beings have ever known or shall ever fathom hereafter.

It is no wonder that many legal battles had ensued with this scientific advancement giving rise to unnatural parenthood.

Perhaps the day is also not far when 'baby deeds' just like 'sale deeds' and 'mortgage deeds' would have to be executed on stamp papers on the basis of some fixed schedule and may also probably require compulsory registration.

Legal Issues of Surrogacy

In legal parlance, any transaction of surrogacy would mean the 'lease' of the carrying mother's body, particularly of her womb, to the parents of the embryo for rearing it to a stage where it becomes a developed child to be handed over at delivery.

Ever since the somewhat recently introduced surrogacy arising out of scientific advancement in modes of natural birth processes has been converted by human ingenuity into a commercial activity, a number of legal issues have cropped up, answers whereof would have to be determined with due regard to provisions of contract and constitutional laws. For clear-cut decisions, it is essential to have a vivid picture of underlying facts and an indepth analysis of the contractual aspects.

The most important question that needs an answer is : is the money consideration being paid to compensate the surrogate for the 'services' rendered, the pains of maternity suffered, or is it towards the purchase of the child? The core of the agreement is truly the child, the services and pains of the accompanying surrogacy being incidental and of no consequence to hirers. No doubt both are unethical as the first one in clear terminology would mean 'womb hiring' and the second alternative amounts to 'baby purchase.' Ethics and morals notwithstanding, the legal issues arising from the subject of surrogacy range from whether the very transaction can at all have a legitimate colouring and if so to determine the respective rights and responsibilities of the hired seller, the surrogate mother *vis-a-vis* the buyer, the genetic parents, as also the duties and responsibilities of the attending physician who play an important role in the entire episode and finally delivers the child and so on.

Broadly speaking, the legal issues involved are:

- should agreements of surrogacy be given a legal recognition or should they be considered void as violating the basic principles of human rights and as being against public policy?
- who should be recognised as legal parents of the child? In *Smith v Jones*,[130] a couple's embryo had been carried by the gestational surrogate. The court considered genetic parents as legal parents and granted them the right to have their names on the birth certificate.
- what would be the genetic mother's stand if the surrogate should change her mind and refuse to part with the baby, even offer to return monetary consideration received? In such cases, should there be a compulsion on the surrogate to part with the baby on delivery and/or should the denial merely lead to monetary

[130]No: 85 53201402 (Michigan Cir Ct, Wayne Co, March 14, 1986) cf. in Keye, Chang, Rebar and Sailes, *Infertility Evaluation and Treatment* 893 (1995) W.B.Saunders & Co.

penalty for breach of contract?

- what would be the duties and liabilities of the doctor in case such agreements are entered into? For example, if the agreement provides that only the genetic parents have the final authority to consent to a Cesarean section, or termination of pregnancy midterm and the doctor finds either of the two necessary in the interest of the surrogate, what would be the validity of the agreement? To whom should he be legally responsible for his act?
- how should monetary compensation received by the surrogate be regarded? Would the contract fall within classification of business? Would the amount be regarded as profits liable to assessment under income tax laws?
- in case a surrogate mother who has already been paid in advance for her services fails to carry the pregnancy full term, would she be liable to return the money for unfulfilled contract, for failure of consideration or for impossibility of performance, or would the compensation be non-refundable?
- if a woman indulges in surrogacy as a 'business' proposition, without the consent of and/or to the displeasure of her husband, what will be his legal remedies?
- what are rights and responsibilities of the surrogate mother if the genetic parents refuse to accept the child after delivery? Still more important: who will be responsible for welfare of such a child in case he is born deformed or handicapped? Do genetic parents have a right to refuse custody in case of abnormality of the child?

These and many more contingencies, one more difficult and heart wrenching than the other, can arise since these issues deal with two sets of human beings and an innocent child who has had no hand in his/her coming into the world artificially through man-made intervention into a divine domain with commercialisation entering into prohibited areas.

With the process becoming more and more common, many countries have introduced regulatory legislation on surrogate motherhood to bring in legality into the abnormal situation. For example, in Arkansas, law itself creates a presumption that the mother of a child conceived by artificial insemination and born to an unmarried surrogate is the intended mother; Arizona legislation grants status of legal mother of the child to the surrogate and, if married, then her husband is presumed to be the legal father; in Florida, the intended parents are presumed to be the legal parents on a determination that at least one intended parent is genetically related to the child, otherwise the woman giving birth is presumed to be the legal mother; New Hampshire and Virginian laws require that a judicial order signed before the pregnancy must vest parental rights to the intended parents.[131]

However, in India, with divergent religions, castes and creeds, where numerous personal laws spell out conflicting legal positions on the same set of facts, with non-existence of a Uniform Civil Code, even formation of legislation would be grossly complex.

Still, with this subject matter getting more complicated, a decision ought to be spelt out for regulating these unusual problems sooner the better. In order to initiate this process, a discussion on some of the legal issues which follow and a study of their implications by an expert committee is surely called for at the earliest.

Surrogacy and Adultery

Whether surrogacy is akin to adultery, as artificial insemination is undertaken with a donor seed and factually the woman bears the child of a man she is not married to.

---

[131] *Ibid.*

Surrogacy and the New Born

The issue of legitimacy of a child born to a surrogate is of utmost importance demanding serious attention of the legislators. Today, fate of the unborn hangs by a delicate thread and depends on many factors like change of mind of one or both of the intended parents or even the surrogate, a possibility of an intervening break in marriage leading to divorce, normalcy or otherwise of an unborn notwithstanding. Some correlated issues also arise: for example, what would be rights of the child with regard to a claim in the share of property of the genetic father? If a couple obtains a divorce before birth of the child, who would be responsible for bringing up the child? Laws concerning such issues generally pivot around the central theme of "welfare of the child" but still utmost clarity is called for as artificiality has entered the arena of nature and natural love and affection that develop between an unborn and the genetic parents during nine months of childbearing have had no chance to develop.

Breach of Contract

A contract involving surrogacy basically revolves around three premises:

- the surrogate offering services to carry the child to term;
- surrogate and her husband (in case she is married), are presumed to have relinquished parental rights upon the signing a contract;
- the amount to be paid to the surrogate by the genetic parents partly in advance and partly at the time of receiving the child in exchange for services rendered.

The validity of such an agreement can be challenged on the ground that:

- it violates principles of human rights;
- it violates statutory requirements as babies are not 'goods';

- it is unethical and contrary to public policy.

Breach of contract of surrogacy could raise some complex and complicated situations. For instance, in case a child is born with some physical deformity and the biological father and his wife refuse to pay the balance of fees agreed upon and/or to adopt the child.

The New Jersey Supreme Court[132] was seized with a matter in which a surrogate mother who, despite a contract to the contrary,[133] refused to part with the baby pleading that it had become a part and parcel of her intrinsic system. Thence ensued a legal tug of war for the custody of the child. The court finally gave custody to the father, with surrogate getting only visitation rights. Incidentally, the court did observe that alternative reproduction methods formed part of the constitutional rights of privacy.[134]

Pro and Anti-surrogacy

The legalists and the moralists are, despite numerous debates, still divided on the desirability or otherwise of surrogacy. The objections of **anti-surrogate legalists** are mainly:

- amounts to commercialisation: Surrogacy, legalised or otherwise, could become a coercive tool in the hands of the

---

[132]M 217 N. J. super 313, 512; 525 A 2ed 1128 (N J Super Ch 1987) Re Baby M, quoted Keye and others, id at 888.

[133]*Id* at 1143. The contract provided the following: Ms Whitehead would assume the risks of pregnancy and childbirth. She would submit to a psychiatric evaluation for which Mr Stern would pay. Mr Stern had the right to name the child.
That in the event of the death of Mr Stern, the child would be placed in the custody of Mr Stern's wife. Mrs Whitehead would not abort the child. In addition she would undergo amniocentesis and if the child were found to have a genetic or congenital abnormality, it would be aborted if Mr Stern requested it.
That in the event the child possessed genetic or congenital abnormalities William Stern would assume legal responsibility for the child once it was born....
Mrs Whitehead was to be paid $ 10,000 and all medical expenses including dental expenses for performing her contractual obligations.

[134]*Ibid.*

wealthy, who would be able to tempt and manipulate the vulnerable and poor sections into renting their organs for monetary benefits ignoring human emotions, physical comfort and domestic viability. This process can lead to an affordable woman hiring younger and poorer ones to carry their babies. In time, 'shopping' for surrogate mothers could become akin to 'shopping' for clothing, furniture and the like;

- the bazaar for "renting of a womb on hire for nine months" is already on the cards with the person paying the rental charges acquiring complete control over the organ rented. It is doubtful whether a surrogate is left with any right to abort the baby even in case of health hazards.

On the other hand, **pro-surrogate legalists** argue that:

- surrogacy has lent hope to childless couples and needs to be encouraged;
- the surrogate, by offering services to carry a child through pregnancy, is not engaging in commerce but is undertaking a noble task;
- the individual's right to have a child is an extension of the right to privacy.

The attack on surrogacy by **anti-surrogate moralists** is based on:

- the procedure amounts to dehumanisation and degradation of women, making them machines of reproduction, which can be hired or purchased temporarily, bringing along a high degree of commercialisation and mechanical reproduction in parenting and undermining the family relations;
- surrogacy is comparable to prostitution whereunder a woman commercialises the use of her body. It is sufficient to cause an emotional trauma to a woman to be deprived of the fruits of

her labour after having carried the child for nine months and suffered pains of childbirth;

- popularisation of this procedure could give rise to an artificial world order leading to marked atheism;
- the entire concept being in defiance of laws of nature would stimulate an unhealthy imbalance in human relationships creating psychological conflicts in offshoots.

The **pro-surrogate moralists** argue:

- love and compassion for humanity are basic pillars on which stands human society. A surrogate must have right to use her own body in the same way as human beings have to donate any other part of their body like their eyes or kidneys.
- recent advancements in medical science have opened up heavens for the otherwise helpless. The pro-surrogates ask, "why should law step in to prevent the helpless from making use of surrogacy which ought to be viewed like transplant of kidneys or hearts. Why should a prospective surrogate be stopped from infusing a ray of hope in the childless couple through this bounty of science?"

Whatever the pros and cons, since surrogacy has entered the portals of society, government must step in and give clear cut indications on the following issues:

Right to Confidentiality

The inevitable intervention of surrogacy in an intimate relationship of a couple, considered in the light of welfare of a child, makes confidentiality in the whole process an essential ingredient. Privacy, in the world of today, is recognised as a basic human right. An ethical responsibility of secrecy founded on the Hippocrates' Oath no doubt does lie on every physician, but it is the surrogate who must abide by the requirement in the interest of the child whom she has nurtured for nine plus months.

Legal intervention is required to fasten accountability on a physician. What would be the liability of a physician for violating the ethical duty of secrecy? Should a physician be liable for compensation by way of damages or should he be made liable for punishment, for example, revocation of licence to practice? The Ohio law provides that a physician maintaining a file "shall not make this information available for inspection by any person" unless a court determines that inspection "is necessary for or helpful in the medical treatment of a child born as a result of artificial insemination."[135]

Records

Medical records to identify all parties involved, the medical and genetic histories of donors and surrogates must compulsorily be maintained by the physician. It may appear beneficial for a physician to provide the following information regarding the donor to a recepient: name, age, height and weight, educational qualifications, religious and caste background, blood group, Rh factor, and the like.

Secrecy does not imply non-maintenance of essential records. Medical records must be maintained, though kept confidential. Data like blood group, specific birth marks, family medical history, allergies etc need to be revealed to the genetic adoptive parents as they are essential for welfare of the child.

Negligence

It is essential for the government to lay down standard base lines on which medical fraternity could operate. Certain basic precautionary requirements must be made mandatory. Reasonable care and caution in carrying out certain procedures would require that only duly qualified physicians should perform these techniques. Contamination of sperms and oocytes must compulsorily be checked

---

[135]Ohio Rev. Code Ann 3111.35(2) (Baldwin) 1987, See Keye and others, *id* at 894.

and transfer of such seeds prohibited and made punishable. The prescribed rules and regulations should be mandatory for medical men dealing with surrogacy and extend to 'acts and omissions' which could affect lives and quality of life of the surrogate and the unborn as that would minimise chances of misutilising these procedures. A paramount duty of the physician is to screen the donor. The importance of a thorough physical examination and blood testing for infectious diseases cannot be over-emphasised as they are the very basic requirements for producing a healthy child. Persons with a family history of malformation, Mendelian disorders or chromosomal derangement should be barred from being donors. Likewise, donors should preferably be free from diseases like asthma, juvenile diabeties mellitus, epileptic disorder, hypertension, psychosis, leucoderma, malignancy and the like, specially those with hereditary trends already confirmed.

Conclusion

Apart from legislation restricting misuse, the medical fraternity as well as social scientists and councillors could be restrained by law from aiding potential vehicles of commercialisation in this arena. Rigorous counselling of women and highlighting the accompanying risk of infection, permanent scarring and other side effects could be introduced at the grassroot levels. Embryo donation must be made a voluntary act without the least trace of coercion or force on either of the partners.

One cannot over emphasise the urgent need for law makers and dispensors of justice to have a basic knowledge of reproductive engineering to enable proper monitoring of the welfare of society. Law makers would require, on one hand, constructive consultations with medical experts and on the other, active public debates before arriving at a workable solution.

If left unchecked by legislation, artificial insemination and surrogate motherhood would, sooner than visualised, lead to a surreptitious market in a new form of flesh trade and an outright invasion on the privacy of the already depressed class, the women. Time is not far when malignant agencies would crop up and engage in trade in women for surrogacy in a full-fledged flesh market thereby escalating immorality, blowing to the winds the noble aim of science.

Today, for good or bad, society has entered a new world order with genetic engineering where methods of reproduction, unknown in the past, are gaining in popularity and becoming common. The ultimate aim of the exercise should of course be to provide a child to the childless parent while ensuring security of the child without inducting commercialisation into this process. Law will have to play a vital role creating rights, imposing duties and settling various disputes that are bound to crop up with such unnatural incursions of medical science into nature's domains and it is necessary that legislation keep pace with a new societal modes. By interaction between lawyers, legal researchers, doctors, social scientists, parents and of course, the judiciary, a *via media* can surely be devised to minimise adverse effects while bestowing advantages of science on the 'needy', in this case, couples wanting to enjoy parenting and perpetuate their family tree.

Yet, let nobility of science not be sullied.

Commercialisation of Human Organs

Rapid advancement in the field of medical science and technology in general, and transplant of human organs saving precious lives in particular, has startled and gladdened the hearts of well-wishers. This surgical excellence has lent a fresh lease of life to those whose flame was to extinguish making doctors the *Messiahs* of a new world order. The transplant system has achieved considerable success in prolonging life or rather, may it be said, defying the call of death for those whose one or other life sustaining organs were diseased, implanting in them a fresh seed of life. An advancement of science over nature again got imprinted on the annals of medical history.

Turmoils and tribulations having escalated in recent times, leading to killings and butcherings, peace has had a sidewalk. The moment some good news gets flashed across the media, the mischief mongers are activated into innovating ways and means of filling their own coffers at the cost of the innocent.

The success of transplant of human organs to save precious lives has given rise to misuse through commercialisation by enticing unwary innocents, mostly the rurals comig to urban areas for medical requirements or the poverty-stricken needy, on to the operation table, relieving them of their organs, often without their knowledge. Mind boggling instances keep on being highlighted by the media but there it ends. Whereas the complacency with which the authorities and citizens are taking these gross violations needs to be strongly condemned, the reports also give out an urgent call for redefining terminologies, framing fresh legislation and implementing it vigorously in order to combat the evil.

Historical Background

The first grains of tissue transplant relate back to five thousand years when early Aryans replaced their noses destroyed by syphilis. Fashion and beauty have always had a great significance for women since the days of Eve. Hindu surgeons were adept at cosmetic operations, in particular, at replacing a nose or an ear.[136]

Records of the more recent times reveal existence of techniques of grafting human tissues dating back to 1875 when Jacques Reverdin, a Swiss surgeon, developed this rare methodology.[137] About a century later, scientists ventured into the field of bone transplants. It was, however, not until 1954 that human kidney transplant was performed by Dr Murray and his colleagues, between identical twins, at the Peter Bent Brigham Hospital at Boston.[138]

Later emerged the era of tissue transplants and then followed bone marrow, intestine, pancreas, livers *et al*. A successful breakthrough for lengthening human life was achieved in 1967 by Professor Christian Bernard, in South Africa, by transplanting a human heart, creating history in sphere of scientific innovations.[139] However, simultaneous with this surgical expertise came the adverse

---

[136]Since having the ear or nose cut off was an accepted form of punishment as well as a common battle injury, this operation was in no way unusual: See, Roderick E. McGrow, *Encyclopaedia of Medical History* 185 (1985) Macmillan Press, London.
[137]*Id* at 329.
[138]Harry Keen, John Jarrett, Arthur Levy, *Triumphs of Medicine* 139 (1976) Paul Elek Ltd.
[139]Dr Tony Smith (ed), *The British Medical Association: Complete Family Health Encyclopaedia* 523 (1996) Dorling Kinderley.

discovery by the almost immediate rejection of the foreign tissue by the recipient body. The results were disappointing, with few patients surviving beyond a couple of months. But the scientists did not lose heart. Further experiments were needed to find out some methodology whereby organ so implanted was accepted by the recipient. Ideas after ideas flooded the scientific mind and further experiments were performed.

A sigh of relief was heaved finally with discovery of the immune suppressant agent, Cyclosporin. Science had again triumphed. Scientists were jubilant. Fresh ideas flooded their ever innovative minds. The process thus begun went on and on. Another marvel paved the way for greater success in organ transplants. The technique of specific donor blood transfusion prior to a living donor organ transplant was developed. These innovations have diminished, rather minimised, the rejection rate of transplanted organs.

Later, in 1969, a team led by Professor Norman Shumway of Stanford University, California, began a programme of heart transplants. By 1984, as many as eighty-five per cent of patients were surviving for at least a year after surgery.[140] The operation was then standardised.

A new era of hope for humankind was visible on the horizon of medical history with transplant of many varied tissues making headway: human organs of the regenerative variety where tissues of the body bear an inherent capacity to replenish themselves offered no difficulty but the non-regenerative part, where on donation the donor loses the vitally functioning organ, loss of which can mean permanent disability or at times even death, spelt a danger zone. In the former variety are included donations of blood, semen and bone marrow while in the latter category stand out kidneys, liver, cornea and the like.

---

[140]*Ibid.*

The very nature of this innovation underlined some logical necessities. A donor of the organ had to be safe-guarded against avoidable adverse effects and pangs of handicap caused by the donation, or else, the very suffering of humankind even for helping another would be undesirable and unethical. Moreover, non availability of organs would itself make the innovation unworkable. The only available source of organs, making the transplants at all viable, were from accident cases or even from persons who had died a natural death, provided organs could be used within a short time post-death as the tissues had to be kept alive for enabling transplant. However, in cases of organs like kidneys, even a living donor could donate one out of two available and still lead a normal life. This required a tremendous coordination and a complete network by hospitals, mortuaries, police, social organisations, donors *et al.* Even with these seemingly unsurmountable hurdles, the new life saving surgeries were gaining ground, in developed and developing countries. In India, the first kidney transplant from a related donor was performed in 1972 at the Christian Medical College, Vellore.

Soon a global market for supply and demand of organs ensued but the supply was still limited and unable to catch up with an ever increasing demand. This imbalance naturally gave rise to marketing of organs as 'goods' and soon a whole community of donors was born. Some of the tissues which got replenished naturally and almost immediately, e.g. blood, became marketable, creating registered blood donor groups. Still non-availability in times of emergencies persisted, for blood donors of the specific matching blood group had to be often tracked and many a time were not available, creating a vaccum for aid to the dying.

In a flash, were invented ways and means for storing blood. This led to establishment of blood banks. The storage was soon taken over by ever ready innovative black-marketeer and a regularised trade in human organ ensued. Soon, illegal, immoral, unethical transactions and clandestine agreements for sale of organs became rampant. The poverty-stricken needy were tempted by greedy middleman to sell one of their kidneys on the premise that human beings could still function normally with the remaining kidney while having sufficient finance to meet his immediate needs. Many came forward voluntarily and willingly to sell their organs. Fathers were found offering their kidney to fulfil dowry demands for their daughters; daughters committed suicide to escape the degradation. As if this was not enough sacrilege on human beings, the assault on human rights soon spread like wild fire, trafficking across the globe, making the underdeveloped economically poor countries scapegoats for feeding organs to rich pasture green lands.

The *modus operandi* led to further demand, kidnapping and forcible removal of organs for sale were added to the nefarious market. Still, the demand surpassed the supply. The prospects of acquiring riches were tremendous and the underworld took over. Question arose: was the scientific intervention, coming between a natural death and possibility of challenging even death, proving to be a boon or a bane for humankind?

Illegal Bandwagon

Global statistics speak loud and clear of unethical elements that have mushroomed in a short span with popularisation of organ transplants. Various wrongful means of dealing with human organs as 'goods' for sale had developed. In fact, under a blanket cover, the supply market of human organs had been flourishing, through a systematised community of agents, subagents and touts ever ready with the goods for a price. In addition, the devil of temptation had stepped in, clouding the receptive minds of the vulnerable, suffering pangs of monetary crunch.

Degrading human organs to marketable commodities, equating them with movable property, regularised trade, targeting the unaffording, luring them with the concept that goods they possessed, their human organs, could be disposed off in a lucrative market for ready cash, were all harming humankind rather than helping the sick. In fact, some went to the extent of even arguing that if it is not an offence for a flat broker to negotiate a flat deal then why should a kidney broker, who does "yeoman service by making two persons, who need each other, meet," be considered an offender?[141] The imbalance between the trader, a manipulative agent, and the donor, in most cases a poor, needy and weak human was too wide. With no restrictive or prohibitive laws to curb this malaise, the temptation swayed, even some doctors, who threw to winds the existing norms and medical ethics by entering the illegal trade.

H Barry Jacobs, a Virginian physician, barred from practice and enamoured by tremendous scope of earnings from sale of organs for transplants, soon established a brokerage company for creating an international market in human organs. The potentiality of profits involved was mind-boggling compared to earnings even in the best of times for one who had practised as a physician. In 1983, as the Medical Director of the million dollar profit making Kidney Exchange Inc, he mailed over seven thousand letters to hospitals soliciting their orders for human organs, tempting citizens of the third world, too well known for their below poverty living conditions, by travel allowance to the United States in addition to an adequate compensation in dollars for loss of one of their kidneys.[142] Flabbergasting examples of the rich exploiting the poor peeped through closed door negotiations but the pathway was illumined as if by a laser beam revealing to the world a twist given to such scientific innovations meant for improving lives of human

---

[141] Per S.B. Jaisinghani, quoted in M.S. Venkataraman "Kidney Donation - Sacrifice or Trade?", *Legal Aspects of Health Care* 172-174 (1995) (Indian Society of Health Administrators).

[142] See Richard B Lillich, "Legal Regulation of the Sale and Transplantation of Human Organs" 2, paper presented at the World Congress on Law and Medicine, Indian Law Institute (New Delhi, 1985).

beings and giving a new lease on life to a few deserving beings.

The project of Jacobs was strongly denounced by medical fraternity in the United States. Despite an acute shortage in availability of human organs, they violently objected to any sort of trade in this sphere. "Immoral and unethical" said The National Kidney Foundation.[143] The American Society of Transplant Physicians, American Society of Transplant Surgeons and International Transplant Society took over the condemnation in a pragmatic and practical way.

Despite such denunciation, back home in India, illegal transactions gained tremendous ground. No legislation governing removal of organs existed. The traders could continue to mint money. Any adult could consent to surgery for removal of any organ. Some unscrupulous elements amongst doctors and others professing to be doctors by displaying faked degrees below their names, began acting as agents themselves and, hand in glove with other agents, recklessly marketed organs and performed surgeries. Sale of kidneys in exchange of ready cash struck a new and compulsive note. 'Kidney for sale' was often the first resort of a poor man to make money and gradually became a readily acceptable modality for tiding over financial crunch in times of need.

Shocking reports began to appear in the media. One report read:

"Government intelligence agencies say India is the world's biggest centre for trade in human organs. The annual turnover in kidneys is estimated to be Rs 40 crore. The trade is also highly organised in cornea, skin and placental tissue. A live kidney costs anything between Rs 30,000 and Rs 1 lakh, a live cornea Rs 80,000 and a patch of skin Rs 1,000."[144]

---

[143] *Ibid.*

[144] *Sunday Observer* (Bombay ed) 5 November 1995.

Another report stated:

"India remains one of the third world's great organ bazaars, with kidney business alone worth Rs 400 million."[145]

The Voluntary Health Association of India confirms illegal business of kidneys is worth Rs.400 million; as kidneys are not available or the patients cannot afford to pay for them, statistics bring out the fact that of the 50,000 transplants required in India, only around 500 are performed officially every year.[146]

Result? Since then innumerable rackets came to be unearthed day in and day out. A major kidney scam involving Turkish patients who had purchased kidneys for price averaging Rs 10 lakhs a piece in Bombay was exposed.[147] Another major kidney racket was unearthed in Bangalore. The story emerged after a twenty-eight year old labourer called Velu visited his doctor and was asked as to why one of his kidneys had been removed. All that he could relate was that he had been lured to a hospital and drugged. He claimed that when he awoke he was told that he had fallen over and needed an operation. He was eventually given rupees five thousand.[148] Bharati Nagar, a grimy slum in Madras suburb of Villivakkam, which has come to be known as 'Kidneyvakkam,' has over a quarter of its two thousand residents surviving on single kidneys.[149] The commission on the finalised deals ranged from Rs 1,000/ to 5,000/. The causes for holding out their organs for sale were multifold. Fathers had sold their kidney to meet the dowry demands for their daughters' marriage; sons had voluntarily deprived themselves of this organ to meet the funeral expenses of their ancestors and so on and so forth.

---

[145] *The Times of India* (Bombay ed) 21 August 1995.
[146] *The Saturday Statesman* (Delhi ed) 15 April 1995.
[147] *Business Standard* (Calcutta ed) 16 April 1995.
[148] *Haj News,* 1 April 1995.
[149] *The Pioneer* (Delhi ed) 24 February 1994.

The issue of removal of organs from live donors, without or with their consent was a horrendous betrayal of human rights. It brought to fore the urgency of a world-wide dialogue on human rights violation, emphasising the need of appropriate legislation to curb 'flesh trade' and the urgency of a campaign for cadaver donations.

Human Rights Perspective

Commercialisation and trade in parts of live human body, the organs, have been held as violative of the recommendations of Universal Declaration of Human Rights, 1948.

Article 1 of the Declaration states :

"All human beings are born free and equal in dignity and rights. They are endowed with reason and conscience and should act towards one another in a spirit of brotherhood."

Articale 3 of the Declation provides :

"Everyone has a right to life, liberty and security of a person."

Article 5 of the Declaration provides :

"No one shall be subjected to torture or to cruel, inhuman or dgrading treatment or punishment."

These Articles were no doubt being grossly violated by tempting, inducing or even ensnaring the poor to part with their body parts takng advantage of their stringent economic conditions or under coercion in order to fulfil the needs and demands of the affluent but then who would intervene? To trade in organs, to buy and sell them for money consideration, has indeed reduced the greatly sanctified human body parts to goods and/or property which can be purchased any time whenever needed and sold to satisfy monetary needs.

There is another potential hazard to human dignity peeping out in the Indian scenario. Availability of human organs for sale creates an inherent fear in the weaker sections that any time they may be compelled to part, advertently or inadvertently, with their own organs to tide over monetary crises, creating general psychological insecurity. The system could also lead to, amongst other crimes, a new mode of matrimonial crimes with husbands and in-laws either compelling the woman to donate her kidney for the benefit of the in-laws family or get the doctor to remove it surreptiously without her knowledge. If wives can be burnt alive for money, why should they be spared when the husband's own family member needs an organs from her? These matters are now coming to the fore and alterations in the existing legislation are already being mooted (discussed later).

The Transplantation of Human Organs Act 1994 - an overview

Rampant uncontrolled increase in illegal organ trade and the pathetic, deft and blood curdling dealings gave rise to necessity of imposing controls, by means of a national legislation, aimed at restricting and punishing illegal transactions with the hope that it might, to some extent, curtail 'dealings' and proliferation of an organ bazaar although such restrictions could boomerang by diminishing considerably the availability of organs to those in need even in times of emergency. However, one had to decide between the devil and the deep sea, non-availability of organs *versus* marketing which had already led to surreptitious exploitation and fraudulent deprival of organs of ignorant unwary and vulnerable poor even by quacks at shady nursing homes.

Bizzare as it surely is, stray cases have occured when taking shelter under such provisions, doctors have succumbed to monetary temptation and in utter disregard of their professional oath and medical ethics as also humanitarian attribute with which every human being is endowed, removed healthy organs without informing either patient or his relatives, sold them to the many agents who ply their trade surreptitiously in the vicinity of hospitals ensnaring innocents on the pretext of taking them to specialists whom they know and who will treat them for such disease from which they may be suffering. Fortunately, such cases of surreptitious organ removals and transplants under cover of secrecy are few and far between and the media has played its role well by quick reporting and highlighting cases that do occur time and again. However, there can be no substitute for severe deterrent punishment for such humans - doctors though they be.

In India, persistent reports of these wide spread human rights violations had put a pressing constraint on Parliament to take effective measures to curb this evil. Thus was passed 'The Transplantation Of Human Organs Act 1994', (hereinafter referred to as the Act). In the first instance, it was brought into force in states of Goa, Himachal Pradesh and Maharashtra and the Union Territories, with an option to other States to adopt the same under clause (1) of Article 252 of the Constitution. The Act was essentially meant to regulate removal, storage and transplantation of human organs for therapeutic purposes, focussing chiefly on methodologies to prevent commercial dealings. Moreover, the entire subject matter was placed in the hands of Appropriate Authorities, Authorisation Committee and registered hospitals and medical practitioners, thus dispensing with quacks and fake nursing homes. This was followed by the passing of The Transplantation of Human Organs Rules, 1995 (hereinafter referred to as the Rules) with a view to regulate the procedures for implementation of the Act.

Live donors apart,the thrust naturally had to fall on ways and means to make organs available from the dead and if they had to be used for therapeutic purposes, then their removal within shortest possible time after 'death.' Thus the thought processes shifted to when a person be declared dead and that led to development of concept of 'brain death' which had already been engaging the minds of scientists for some time.

The Indian Penal Code nowhere defined death or evaluated its concept. However, Registration of Birth and Death Act, 1969 defines death to mean, "when all life ceases." The Harvard criteria originally postulated four characteristics of brain death: "unreceptivity and unresponsiveness to externally applied stimuli and internal needs; no spontaneous movement or breathing; no reflex activity; a flat electro encephalograph reading after a 24 hours period of observation."[150]

These definitions came under active re-consideration because of the urgency accompanying removal of life saving organs from the dead and their immediate use for therapeutic purposes. *Prima facie*, the medical fraternity appeared to be unanimous that when the brain dies, the ventilator takes over lung functions, and the body, as a whole, ceases to be functional. However, mistakes in diagnosis are not impossible, or even uncommon, utmost caution has to be exercised in each and every case before certifying death.

The Act recognised and brought to the fore few existing concepts vital to any legislation dealing with rights of human beings e.g. consent and brain stem death. In consonance with the objects of the Act, sources for availability of organs were as if divided into two categories: those from dead and from living human beings. However, consent of a donor is the golden thread that runs throughout the Act as the key-note for such removal.

Thus rules and regulations for removal of human organs from the dead require his consent, given before his death,[151] or that of his near relatives,[152] after his death,[153] provided the deceased person had not objected to the removal even after death during his life time.

---

[150]L.M. Singhvi. "Need to Redefine Concept of Death", *Times of India* (Bombay ed) 24 Feb 1992.
[151]Ss. 3 (1) and (2) Act, See Appendix A-Part D.
[152]S. 2 (i), *id.*
[153]S. 3 (3), *id.*

In keeping with the jurisprudential notion of consent, technically, any person, who has completed age of 18 years,[154] can voluntarily authorise removal of any of his organs[155] for transplant[156] for therapeutic purposes.[157] An old man or woman can also donate his/her organs. While age is the apparent criterion for eligibility, mental condition of a donor is of utmost importance. Thus an insane person who is incapable of understanding the nature and consequences of his act of authorising removal of his organ is excluded from the purview of eligibility. In this context, Indian Contract Act makes it clear that those persons who have reached age of majority and those who are of sound mind and are not particularly disqualified from contracting by any law to which they are subject, are competent to contract.[158]

The Act sought to place restrictions even on giving/taking of consent for removal of organs from donors for recipients. Thus, no organ can be removed from body of a donor before his death and transplanted into a recipient unless donor is a near relative of the recipient.[159] In other cases, i.e. where donation is claimed to be out of affection or attachment to the recipient, prior approval of Authorisation Committee constituted under the Act is a must.[160]

In the absence of consent, and that too given under conditions and in such manner prescribed under the Act, removal of organ from a live person would amount to 'voluntary causing grievous hurt'* attracting punishment under penal laws.

An exception to this blanket prohibition lies in authorisation

---

*See Glossary.

[154]S. 2 (f), *id.*

[155]S. 2 (h), *id.*

[156]S. 2 (p), *id.*

[157]S. 2 (o), *id.*

[158]S. 11, Indian Contract Act: See Appendix A-Part A.

[159]S. 9 (1), Act: see Appendix A-Part D.

[160]S. 9 (3), *id.*

under section 92 of the Penal Code[161] where, in case of emergencies, a doctor can remove an organ without consent in circumstances wherein it is impossible for a patient to signify consent, or if that patient is incapable of giving consent and, there is no guardian or other person with lawful charge of the sufferer capable of giving consent. Even in such a contingency, it is essential that removal of organ must be for the benefit or interest of the patient. In such cases, a doctor assumes temporary guardianship and acts under a legal cloak, conditionally, in 'good faith' and with 'due care and attention,'* for the 'benefit'* of the patient. In such a case, the objective, is not to obtain organ for sale or use otherwise but only to save, or to improve quality of life, of a patient.

Due to a wave of commercialisation of organs that had swept the country by storm, not only legal barriers were erected to curb the evil, a severe responsibility was also clamped on registered medical practitioner[162] who was to carry on the invasion. Thus, before removing an organ from a live person, he has to ensure that the donor: has duly authorised removal of his organ; has given free and informed consent; is in a proper state of health and medically fit to be subjected to procedure of organ removal; that recipient is a near relative of the donor for which also a few confirmatory tests are mandatory.[163] In case recipient is a spouse of the donor, it would be necessary to record a statement to that effect.[164] In case the donor or the recipient claim that donation of organ is out of affection or attachment to the recipient, the matter has to be referred to an Authorisation Committee constituted under the Act, for prior approval.[165] In fact, the Union Health Ministry is considering exclusion of 'spouse' and inclusion of 'grandparents' as it is feared

*See Glossary.

[161]S. 92, see Appendix A - Part B.

[162]S. 2 (n): see Appendix A-Part D.

[163]R. 4 (1) (c): see Appendix A - Part E.

[164]R. 4(1) (d) and Form 4, *id.*

[165]*Supra* n 160.

that there is a strong possibility of rejection in such cases as also a probability of undue pressure to compel a woman to donate, against her will, to her husband. The exclusion of foreign nationals is also under active consideration in order to check dealings for commercial gains.[166]

In the United Kingdom, The Human Tissues Act 1961,[167] regulates use of human organs of dead for therapeutic purposes. It also provides for bequests by a person desirous of donating his organs after his/her death. In consonance with English legislation, in India also, the authorisation has to be made in the presence of two witnesses. However, taking into account prevalent illiteracy of masses, and the fact that rampant illegal transactions and surreptitious commercialisation had already taken deep roots, it has been provided that at least one of the witnesses to the authorisation should be a near relative of the donor. Also, whereas the English legislation provides for the bequest by a terminally ill person, the Indian counterpart is wider and permits 'any person' to make such a bequest.

In India, limited donation of organs by will is traced by psychologists to a long-standing mental aberration whereby making a will is looked upon as a precursor of death. Few humans like to face reality, or to think of death and plan for it. Therefore, signing papers for removal of organs post-death, arouses at times, for those afraid of the thought of their end, the worst type of fear syndrome which prevents them from even considering it, much less to proceed

---

[166] *The Hindu* (New Delhi ed.) 12 August 1997.

[167] Section 1(1) of the Act states: "If any person, either in writing at any time or orally in the presence of two or more witnesses during his last illness, has expressed a request that his body or any specified part of his body be used after his death for therapeutic purposes or for the purposes of medical education or research, the person lawfully in possession of the body after his death may, unless he has reason to believe that the request was subsequently withdrawn, authorise the removal from the body of any part or, as the case may be, the specified part, for use in accordance with the request."

with the formalities.

In case of removal after death of a person, a duty is cast on the medical practitioner to ensure: that the donor has, before death, unequivocally authorised organ removal in presence of two or more witnesses; at least one of whom is a near relative of the deceased; that there was no subsequent revocation of aforesaid authorisation and lastly that removal was for therapeutic purpose.[168]

A more stringent requirement to be observed before removal of any organ from the body of a deceased person which is mandatory for the doctor is to ensure by means of clinical examination that life of the person is extinct.[169] However, in the case of brain-stem death,[170] certification by a board of medical experts is prescribed by law as a mandatory requirement.[171] The medical panel thus set up is required to certify that the person "is dead on account of permanent and irreversible cessation of all functions of the brain-stem."[172]

In the case of brain-stem death occurring in a person who is less than 18 years of age, after medical certificate as required above is obtained, parents of such a person may authorise removal of organs for therapeutic purpose.[173] Besides, a doctor is duty-bound to determine that organs being removed are in a fit state for removal and transplant.

In case of dead bodies lying in a hospital or prison and not claimed for 48 hours, from the time of death, by any near relative of the deceased person, organ removal is to be authorised by the in-charge of management and control of hospital or prison or by an

---

[168]R. 4 (2): see, Appendix A-Part E.
[169]S. 3 (5): see, Appendix A-Part D.
[170]S 2 (d), *id.*
[171]S. 3 (6) *id* and Rule 4(3) (a).
[172]Form 8, Rule and Brain Stem Death Certificate annexed to Form 8 of Rules.
[173]R. 4 (3) (b) and Forms 8 and 9 Rules: see Appendix A-Part E.

employee of such hospital or prison authorised in this behalf by a person in charge of management or control.[174]

Also such authorisation is barred if a person having authority to release the body for removal of organs has "reason to believe that any near relative of the deceased person is likely to claim the dead body even though such near relative has not come forward" within the specified time.[175]

In case of bodies sent for post-mortem examination for medico-legal reasons, where death has occurred due to accident or any other unnatural cause, or for pathological purposes, a competent person may authorise removal of organs for therapeutic purposes if he has reason to believe that human organ will not be required for further post-mortem proceedings. In such cases, it is also essential to ensure that the deceased had not, during his lifetime, objected to his organs being used for therapeutic purposes after his death.[176]

However, consequences of legislative curbs have been non-availability of organs when needed the most. Therefore, some via-media solutions appear to be the call of the day for which think-tanks need to be put into action. In search of other avenues, it has been argued that to meet growing demands of organs for transplant and to improve upon availability in times of necessity, legislation should permit removal of organs from the deceased, irrespective of consent and regardless of consent of relatives. There are many arguments against such a proposition. If right to life guaranteed under the Constitution of India could be interpreted as right to death,[177] then right to live with human dignity[178] could also possibly be extended to right to die with dignity. To stand on one's dignity

---

[174] S. 5 (1) : Appendix A-Part D.
[175] S. 5 (2), *id.*
[176] S. 6, *id.*
[177] *P Rathinam Nagbhusan Patnaik v Union of India,* AIR 1994 SC 1844.
[178] *Francis Coralie v Delhi Administration,* AIR 1981 SC 746.

is defined as "to demand to be treated with proper respect."[179] On the one hand, removal could be justified on the ground of saving human lives; on the other, to trespass on wishes and mutilate the corpse by removal of organs in supercessian of the wishes of the deceased or his/or her relatives would amount to indignity as well as infringement of human sentiments. Which in a country like India is indeed unthinkable.

Even a debate on this suggestion can raise issues of legal and ethical significance. Would it be an infringement of human rights? Would it be a curb on freedom of an individual? Does State have a right to play with the feelings of the bereaved in times of their utmost grief? Would such a step be in consonance with the socialistic pattern of society? To make matters worse confounded, some religions have mandates against tampering with body parts. According to Christianity, organ removal is not consistent with provisions of body resurrection.[180]

Therefore, considering hurdles in closing in from the other end by creating a legal compulsion that organs shall be removed from dead for the ultimate benefit of the living, a possible *via media* would be to permit such removal unless specifically prohibited by deceased during his lifetime. It is probable that this kind of a provision would at least act as a compulsion on persons to record their wills (and incidentally, objections to removal of their organs after death) during their life time.

Striking a golden mean, it can be affirmed that suggestions favouring such pathways are not worth debating and need to be shelved without further thought.

---

[179]See, *supra* n 48, at 374.

[180]The sixth canon enacts, amongst other things, that clerks shall not inflict or order to be inflicted mutilation of a limb on any persons whomsoever: See, Smith William, *Christian Antiquities* 244, vol 1 (1875) John Murray, London.

Ban on Removal of Organs

The Act bans removal of organs from body of the deceased person if there is "reason to believe that an inquest may be required to be held in relation to such body in pursuance of provisions of any law for the time being in force."[181] In any case, those entrusted with the body "solely for purpose of interment, cremation or other disposal" cannot authorise removal.[182]

Preservation of Human Organs

The Act does not prescribe or sanction any particular method for preservation of organs but has left the scope wide by stating that organs shall be preserved "according to current and accepted scientific methods in order to ensure viability for the purpose of transplantation."[183]

Restrictions on Removal and Transplantation of Human Organs

Under the Act, Central Government and State Governments have been authorised to constitute one or more Authorisation Committees for smooth implementation of the restrictions that may be placed by respective governments.[184] The Committee is empowered to reject applications made by prospective donors and recipients for which reasons have to be recorded in writing.

Regulatory Provisions

In order to effectively deal with the restrictions and curbs placed on removal and transplant of human organs, the Act has made it mandatory for hospitals to register in case of their being involved in the relevent procedures.

The Act also deals with appointment of Appropriate

---

[181]S. 4 (1), Appendix A-Part D.
[182]S. 4(2), *id.*
[183]R. 5: see, Appendix A-Part E and S. 7 Act: see, Appendix A-Part D.
[184]S. 9 (4) (a) & 9(4) (b) Rules: see, Appendix A-Part E.

Authority by Central and State Governments, functions of the Authority, registration of hospitals,[185] including issuance of certificate for registration,[186] and the suspension and/or cancellation of registration.[187]

Penal Liabilities

The Act prescribes imprisonment upto a term of five years and fine upto rupees ten thousand in case of persons indulging in organ transplant without authority.[188] In case any person is convicted under the Act, and such person happens to be a registered medical practitioner, his name is reported to the State Medical Council for action including removal of his name from the register of practitioners for a period of two years for the first offence and permanently in case of repetition of offence.[189]

By way of abundant caution, it is further provided that the court would have to state its reasons in the judgment in case it decides to impose a sentence or fine less than the minimum prescribed.[190] Considering barbaric intrusion into human body by the ones who are expected and licensed to treat diseases rather than harm sufferers, that too surreptitiously, throwing moral and medical ethics to winds, and in the process belittling the services of the medical profession, the punishment prescribed appears to be rather lenient.

Conclusion

Saving of lives through organ transplant was indeed a scientific miracle, the scientists' gift to humanity. In today's advanced era, with efforts being made to curb sickness and disease, achieve

---

[185]S. 14 Act: see, Appendix A-Part D.
[186]S. 15, id.
[187]S. 16, id.
[188]S. 18(1), id.
[189]S. 18 (2), id.
[190]S. 19, id.

longevity for humankind, it is but natural that this innovation should have caught up the world in a big way, not only amongst affluent but also the not so affording middle class. However, what was intended to be a boon, unfortunately caught the evil eye of the underworld dons, specially of developed countries, leading to serious exploitation of poor sections in the underdeveloped nations creating a flourishing market in human organs.

Nothing being more precious than the spark of life, when a near and dear one is suffering and the relatives know that the life ebbing away could be saved, if only another human being's organs could be transplanted in place of the diseased one, they are willing to go to any extent to get a miraculous life-saver. The poverty-stricken bread-feeder of a large family, father of a marriageable daughter caught in the net of a dowry demand, the purely greedy human being and many more such vulnerable sections abound in poor under-developed countries and thus have the intermediaries been ruling the roost since decades. Demand-supply ratio and more so the acute emergency demand *vis-a-vis* immoral greedy underworld suppliers, have led to a commercial crime-infested market where not only those willing to sell their organs are exploited to their very bones, but many hale and hearty persons, specially children, are kidnapped and put under the knife and next day, victims minus the organ that is surreptitiously removed for sale, are left outside hospitals or on the wayside to fend for themselves.

It is too late in the day to go into the reverse gear and stop transplants altogether on the ground that, while proving to be a blessing to quite a few affluents, the system has adversely affected weaker sections of society, for today, demand for organs has achieved tremendous boost and is as if woven into the warp and weft of society. Total prohibitory measures applied could mean a death sentence to some of the precious lives which could probably be saved and in practical politics, will merely increase the black-market value to astronomical heights.

Yet, nature sees to it that innovations and successes fall into the lap of those who work dedicatedly. If one door is closed, science and scientists quickly move towards others and fresh avenues are opened earlier than can be visualised.

The Batista operation, a radical procedure that could help heart patients avoid transplants, was tried out for the first time in India, at the Institute of Cardiovascular Diseases run by Madras Medical Mission. The impugned operation was performed on a 28 year old woman who had been kept waiting for months for availability of a heart for transplant but was saved by this new alternative mode. The second one followed in quick succession and was performed on a 36 year old patient who had been close to death for want of a donor heart.[191]

Had there been an easy-availability of hearts for transplant, this wonder innovation may not have seen the light of the day for ages. However, the dedication of scientists has always come to the rescue of humankind. Medical scientists have been consistently improving on modes leading to health and longevity for man and are still working ceaselessly to benefit in every way. It is, therefore, for us and the administrators to aid them by devising suitable machinery for putting their success to fruitful use and not as a tool to exploit the poor, converting boons to curses. Today, it has become essential to focus on underworld dons and their misdoings and 'dot tight' and 'money proof' administration to put them to use as intended.

Apart from laws and an efficient machinery for enforcing them, it is also necessary to have deterrant measures. Where punishment is tardy, crime abounds. Therefore, laws must provide severe penalties for those who indulge in crime of ruining and mutilating live human-beings without their consent and/or active

[191]G V Krishnan, "Batista Operation helps make the failing heart a better pump," *The Times of India* (Bombay ed) 26 November 1996.

participation merely for the sake of filling their palatial mansions with gunny-bags of wealth.

More essential is the quick and efficient, ruthless and electrifying punishment to the guilty, whatever be the chair occupied and the power it is supposed to wield. If the occupiers have soiled the sacred chairs, they ought to be dealt with as criminals and not as power-lords. The politician-criminal nexus has harmed the nation and its poverty-stricken masses to no end and it is high time this crime infected era is brought to a close.

More important than legislation and human rights protection organisations are the processes and programmes for mass education and quick forceful enlightenment of each and every citizen on specific subjects which are harming them most. More essential than even mass enlightenment through education which is indeed time consuming and challenging, is to awaken Indian masses from their fatal complacency and make them aware of their rights as human beings.

In the present context, it is for citizens and rulers to rise against violation of basic human rights, refuse malafide intervention of money-lords and stop surreptitious introduction of commerce into sacred arena of human lives by illegal and fraudulent methods. A mass movement on the lines of India's fight for freedom can still change the grimy scenario of today to a bright future for truly needy sick lives.

Even so, no enactment can serve its purpose if its provisions are neither read nor understood, neither respected nor implemented by the medical fraternity who must constantly update their knowledge and honour the trust placed in them by patients. Gone are the days when doctors could afford to remain unaware of legal provisions and procedures and lawyers ignorant of human anatomy. They are the ones on whom lies a two-pronged responsibility of the masses and to whom every human being turns in their times of stress and strain or even disaster.

Factually speaking, after The Human Organ Transplant Act came into force, doctors and hospitals put their tools down and not a single transplant had been performed in Mumbai for a long time. Finally, when a case did come up at the Hinduja Hospital in May 1996, the surgery was not performed because of confusion as to who was to authorise it.[192] This is where doctors could come into the picture as samaritans of a high order. If only they rise above the rest, keep abreast with medico-legal updates and refuse to soil their hands in murky deals, agents, traders and underworld dons will soon abandon their prestigious posts and disappear from the scenes where poor needy sick could have been exploited and usher in an era when the sick would be treated as sick irrespective of their money strings and cared for like human beings in need of care.

The best medicine for humankind today is : let law and medicine correlate to become *Messiahs* of the masses and missiles for crime.

[192]The Times of India (Bombay ed) 15 November 1996.

Role of A Doctor in Case of Road Accident

The twentieth century has witnessed global revolutionisation of the automobile industry. An indication of increasing prosperity, with its many advantages, has also brought inevitable harm to humanity caused by environmental pollution and increased road accidents, resulting in loss or impairment of many a human life or limb. Recent wave of liberalised economy in India, without any pre-thinking to infrastructural facilities, has claimed many lives and limbs with the upsurge in road accidents, putting authorities and medical personnel under a severe strain.

On the one hand, unbridled affluency of a few with phenomenal increase in the number of cars and their sizes has garnered a serious challenge to the traffic. To add to the chaos, have been introduced scooters, motorcycles, autorickshaws and the like for the benefit of large middle class. On the other hand, are poverty-stricken rurals, migrating to urban areas in thousands each day, squeezed like sardines in public transport to reach their destination, the haven that is supposed to feed and clothe them, leading to an inevitable increase in a number of public transport vehicles, all together creating confusion, chaos and challenging road situations with increasing number of accidents, leaving in their trail dead and/ or battered humans.

Considering the seriousness of the situation, it is high time projects and programmes for inculcating road safety habits in the young, right from stage of nursery, when material dispositions intertwine with formed habits to pave their paths in new lives, are introduced by every State. Various other measures like propagating effects of rash driving, or while under the influence of alcohol, also need to be introduced. Many more stringent measures like keeping non-road worthy vehicles off roads, introducing harsher rules for issue of learner's licences, weeding out graft from the process of issuing confirmed licences, enforcing an upper and lower age limit for drivers, strict supervision and cross check of medical certificates, enforcing minimum educational qualifications for practitioners authorised to issue such certificates, and above all, a deterrent punishment to the wrong doer and implementing them scrupulously may lead to controlling road accidents to some extent. Not the least important aid would be that of developing and maintaining better roads, constructing parapets in danger zones like mountainous regions and *ghats*, etc. One can then hope to safeguard human lives and limbs and reduce the menace to some extent.

In the days gone by, road accidents were attributed to either ill luck or perhaps to divine wrath. A little later, with advent of mechanised transport on the scientific scenario, when vehicles paved their paths onto the roads, accidents were clamped onto the failure of machinery rather than ill-fate or destiny. However, in the face of a stress dominated life of the common man today, with psyche of man controlling the machine determining his style of driving, with reckless young of *nouveau*-rich class getting addicted to driver's seat, and liberalised economic policies adding new and still newer tempting models with hectic speed on the roads, there has been a spurt in road accidents with statistics flashing flabbergasting figures like:

> "more than eighty crore vehicles (including fifty crore cars) are at any given moment speeding away or struggling in traffic

jams. To add to the chaos, four hundred and fifty lakh new vehicles are being manufactured every year. With a growth in the human population of nine crore a year, the arrival of two new babies is accompanied by the arrival of one new vehicle."[193]

In India, the incidence of road accidents is indeed heart-wrenching. Though India's motor vehicle population accounts for only one per cent of the world's, its share in road accidents is almost six per cent; there is an accident every two minutes, and a death every ten minutes, the pedestrians and two wheeler riders being most vulnerable in metropolitan cities.[194] Deteriorating conditions reveal the increasing pressure on the medical man in relation to road accidents.

The doctor, playing a preventive as well as therapeutic and compassionate role, is the key player in the case of road accidents. He comes into the picture, firstly, with a crucial responsibility, at the time of issuing learner's licence which requires a compulsory medical check-up. He could, by issuing a certificate inadvertently, be responsible for causing a number of accidents which otherwise might have been averted. On the other hand, he could also, by strict scrutiny of the medical condition, restrict to a large extent the issuance of those licences which could indirectly harm even his beneficiaries. Though this role of the medical man may not appear to be directly correlated to road accidents, yet it is a doctor who could greatly influence, if not control, its statistics.

However, once an accident does occur, doctor is the most 'wanted' human being and the earlier his services are made available, and quicker he is installed as the master of ceremonies, greater the chances of saving a human life involved or at least giving succour to the injured. It is said that first hour after the accident, referred to as 'golden hour,' is of great importance during this phase. Therefore,

---

[193]Dr P S Pasricha, *You Only Live Once* 1 (1995) Nasha Publication, Mumbai.
[194]*Ibid.*

immediate emergency post-accident intervention is the most pressing challenge that a doctor has to face in case of road accidents.

An incidental role that he has to play in this field is when he is called upon to discharge his duties as a medical witness in criminal prosecutions or in civil proceedings.

This chapter deals with role of a doctor, not as a driver of the vehicle which *per* chance encounters a road accident in which case he would be treated as any other citizen but rather his role as a medical person, his responsibilities in issuance of medical certificates, his rights and responsibilities *vis-a-vis* moral obligations in treatment of accident victims, and his inevitable role as an expert witness* in medico-legal litigation.

Medical Fitness Certificate

For a person applying for a learner's licence, a medical fitness certificate, from a registered medical practitioner, who is to certify the applicant's physical and mental capacity/incapability, is mandatory.[195] The doctor's opinion decides whether he/she is physically fit[196] to undertake driving so that a licence may be granted. However, and rather surprisingly though, it is the applicant alone, and not a medical practitioner who certifies whether he/she

*See Glossary.

[195]Ss. 8(3) and (4) Motor Vehicles Act, 1988: see, Appendix A-Part F.

[196]In short, the doctor has to satisfy himself that the applicant:

*does not suffer from any defect of vision or that the defect stands corrected by suitable glasses;

*can distinguish pigmentary colours, specifically red and green;

*is able to distinguish with his eye sight at a distance of 25 meters in good day light a motor car number plate;

*does not suffer from a degree of deafness which would prevent his hearing the ordinary sound signals;

*does not suffer from night blindness;

*does not suffer from any defect or deformity or loss of limb which would interfere with the efficient performance of his duties as a driver.

See Form 1-A, Medical Certificate annexed to Form 2 for Grant or Renewal of Learner's Licence.

is suffering from any specific disease, or from epilepsy, or any sudden attacks of loss of consciousness or giddiness from any cause.[197]

In this age of scientific advancement and specialisation, it is unfortunate that rules and regulations for certifying suitability or otherwise of applicants for driving have stagnated in their antique form, necessitating fresh thinking and updating of these legal requirements. A medical practitioner cannot be expected to find out the existence of ailments arising from mental disorders, epilepsy,* etc, in a single check-up unless he is specifically equipped with medical history of the examinee and possesses an infrastructure for basic investigations, for example, equipment for electrocardiogram or an x-ray invasion. The visual and auditory examination, being the two senses which are most crucial for driving could be adjudged best by ophthalmologists and ear specialists, those professionally skilled in the respective fields, who are also equipped with sophisticated paraphernalia for proper examination. To expect a general practitioner to embark upon the domain of the specialist defeats the very object of prescribing an examination and certificates of fitness.

It is therefore suggested that the licensing authority should constitute an approved panel of medical experts from various specialities for conducting a detailed examination prior to issuance of a fitness certificate which would form the main baseline for driving licences entitling a person to sit at the wheel. Of course, every stringent law leaves in its trail a number of loopholes and marginal provisions which negate good by bad. Even today, reportedly, in some places, licence can be acquired without even going for a driving test or a medical examination, only through money power. In case an applicant qualifies for the 'influential category,' then perhaps even 'money' could be omitted. However, keeping a check

[197]Form 1, Application-cum-Declaration as to physical fitness annexed to Form 2 for Grant or Renewal of Learner's licence.

on these fraudulent modes, prescribing more stringent punishment for lapses and an effective mode for prosecution could possibly contain the existing menace to some extent.

The real contribution of medical science in prevention of motor accidents, specially with expanding knowledge of psychology, would be achieved if one could demarcate an 'accident prone' personality, so that they be not only rejected for licence but also educated not to even attempt the wheel. This might require an organised setting up of a series of physiological and psychological tests, including personality determination tests, to designate the applicants as either 'fit for licence' variety or 'accident prone' ones. However, although research scientists have attempted to define very many mysterious personality disorders with descriptive terms ranging from aggressive, insecure, maladjusted, inconsistent, excessively hostile, and so on *ad infinitum*, they have also cautioned that every single individual could possibly be saddled with one or more of the attributes. It cannot be gainsaid that if such criterion was to be enlisted as disqualification, may be, not one individual could safely be certified as fit to get a licence. This is where failure of the tests has finally resulted in their inconclusive finale in the past.

If scientists ever succeed in solving the mystery of demarcating accident prone personality, it would perhaps be their greatest contribution towards prevention of road accidents. Hopefully, with research being conducted in this regard, some well tested battery of personality tests to screen those whose personality profiles fit into the description of a typical 'accident prone' variety may soon see the light of the day and one may then optimistically look forward to diminishing the accident menace. Of course, how viable a proposition such a test would be in the Indian scenario, bearing in mind the economics of the venture, is a different matter altogether and quite outside the purview of the doctor's role. Also, the conclusiveness of this test would itself be required to be put to test for a few years before striking a positive note for, indeed, if the declared 'accident prone' variety in reality encounter lesser accidents than those not so diagnosed, but rather used to driving when drunk, then the entire utility of the test would be brought to a low ebb.

Post-accident Medical Care

Once a road accident occurs, first essential would be to provide emergency first aid to the victim of the accident. For this, it is essential to improve emergency medical services. In fact, it is the first hour following an accident, referred to as the 'golden hour,' which can save the life of many, given instant medical aid. In the United States, emergency helicopters are pressed into service, at various platforms, to lift victims, with the result that, within minutes, the injured are lifted with expert care to the nearest hospital where they get immediate medical aid. Unfortunately, medical emergency set up in India is not yet monitored to meet the needs of the victim during the initial phase or may be even thereafter to any effective levels with the result that, quite often, victims of accidents simply groan away in pain or die before any aid reaches them. Also, it is a known fact that many passers by or those who witness an accident deliberately turn a blind eye, not because they are not compassionate human beings, not willing to help those in need, but, because they do not want to get entangled into subsequent police interrogations and waste of their precious time in today's antiquated legal system.

Today, factually, doctors prefer to direct the injured to hospitals equipped with medico-legal infrastructure although in so doing precious life-saving moments are lost, many a times resulting in the victim succumbing to injuries.

In a public interest litigation brought before Supreme Court of India,[198] Their Lordships have observed:

"No law or State action can intervene to avoid/delay the

---

[198] *Supra* n 93.

discharge of the paramount obligation cast upon members of the medical profession. ...Zonal regulations and classifications cannot also operate as fetters in the process of discharge of the obligation and irrespective of the fact whether under instructions or rules, the victim has to be sent elsewhere or how the police shall be contacted, the guideline indicated in the 1985 decision of the Committee on Forensic Medicine (set up by the Ministry of Home Affairs of the Government of India),[199] is to become operative."[200]

With judicial system being what it is, at times, the attending doctor is called upon to remain present in the court on several dates of hearing and is made to wait till the case is finally called out or adjourned. No reputed doctor with any practice worth his name,

---

[199]The Committee under the Chairmanship of the Director-General of Health Services ...had taken the following decisions:
1. Whenever any medico-legal case attends the hospital, the medical officer on duty should inform the Duty Constable, name, age, sex of the patient and place and time of occurence of the incident, and should start the required treatment of the patient. It will be the duty of the Constable on duty to inform the concerned police station or higher police functionaries for further action.
Full medical report should be prepared and given to the police, as soon as examination and treatment of the patient is over. The treatment of the patient would not await for the arrival of the Police or completing the legal formalities.
2. Zonalisation as has been worked out for the hospitals to deal with medico-legal cases will only apply to those cases brought by the police. The medico-legal cases coming to the hospital of their own (even if the incident has occurred in the zone of other hospital) will not be denied the treatment by the hospital where the case reports, nor the case will be referred to other hospital because the incident has occurred in the area which belongs to the zone of any other hospital. The same police formalities as given in para 1 above will be followed in these cases.
All Government Hospitals, Medical Institutes should be asked to provide the immediate medical aid to all the cases irrespective of the fact whether they are medico-legal cases or otherwise. The practice of certain Government institutions to refuse even the primary medical aid to the patient and referring them to other hospitals simply because they are medico-legal cases is not desirable. However, after providing primary medical aid to the patient, patient can be referred to other hospital if the expertise facilities required for the treatment are not available in that institution.

[200]Supra n 93, at 2043.

would intentionally enter the hornet's nest where his self-respect and time are not valued. Unless these conditions are drastically improved by the higher administrative machinery of government and satisfactory arrangements for recording of evidence of medical man introduced, very few doctors, if any, would willingly attend on accident victims.

There is an immediate need to enforce ways and means for promoting emergency medical services, perhaps in the form of an effective network, where the services of several non-government organisations could be called into play to take up the task of aiding accident victims as their social service oriented projects. Although efficiently run helicopter services may be a far cry, at least quick and efficient ambulance services can be made available at traffic aid posts and police booths, fitted with wireless and telephone facilities, equipped with first aid so as to establish an efficient co-ordination between the police control room and the ambulance service. The more organised the set up, the more effective would be the first aid imparted to the victims of road accidents.

The drivers of public transport system which fill to capacity nearly all public roads and highways have a key role to play in this regard. The most effective mode of providing quick aid to the victims would be to make training in first aid mandatory for the drivers and conductors of public transport vehicles at the very inception of their service. Also, imparting skills of temporary immobilisation of fractured limbs so as not to cause more harm to the victim in the process of transport, in social engineering systems and realisation of the good they would be doing to society at large by acquiring competency in this social welfare schemes would help. To introduce a compulsive note, a certificate of medico-social training could be made mandatory for a licenced driver to get absorbed as riders of public transport vehicles. First aid kits should be made available in all coaches which ply on the highways as well as of city public transport vehicles including taxis and autorickshaws. Immediate incentives to drivers of public transport like taxis and autorickshaws, who help by transporting the accident victims to the nearest hospital, can also be introduced.

No safety devise of public interest is as important as of containing drivers and conductors of contract bus organisations and school buses.

A key role in first aid can be played by police officers and those manning 'road safety patrol' who need to be well equipped with their kits to render help to victims in distress and also possess facilities like wireless, to intimate immediately the occurrence of an accident to nearest medical aid centre to be in readiness to receive an emergency patient if at all life of the victim is to be saved. Today, practically speaking, plight of an accident victim is as pitiable as it is damaging. Either the victim lies by the road side for hours on end, bleeding and groaning, or is huddled into a vehicle so recklessly that, in all probability, it would dislocate an undislocated joint, further compound a fracture or damage the delicate nervous system. These 'secondary accidents' need to be avoided by resorting to adequate training in first aid and correct methods of transportation.

If the victim is found unconscious, simple measures like turning the patient and placing him in a semi-prone position so as to aid respiration, increases victim's chances of survival; for if the victim is lying flat on the back, the tongue may fall backwards and suffocate him. It may be even essential to pull out the tongue and clean it of dirt or debris depending on the extent of post-accident damage. At times artificial respiration or closed chest cardiac massage can save a patient's life, even if no pulse is felt. Splinting of a fractured limb in order to maintain it in an optimal position, while the patient is being transported to the nearest medical aid centre or hospital, is essential. For example, the injured leg may be tied to the sound leg, the injured finger may be tied to a sound one, so on and so forth. These are the easiest methods of splintage. However simple, these measures if taken within minutes can save many an accident case from fatal or damaging consequences. These methods are often most simple requiring the least paraphernalia but the basics should be clear and the methods known.

Probably, some system could be introduced whereby a rescuer is not detained at the police station or a government or a municipal hospital. The life of the victim being of paramount importance and each moment lost being precious, the procedures of *panchnama** and all other formalities should be such that precious minutes, of the victims as well as willing helpers, are not lost. It is therefore essential that rules, regulations and minimum requirements of laws should be systematically flashed through media as part of a literacy campaign.

Morally speaking, it ought to be the concern of every person to come to aid of another human being in distress. However, for a medical person it is a call of duty to rush to a victim to give him benefit of his skill and training, however, lengthy time consuming procedures and implications which follow, have prompted doctors to avoid, as far as possible, accident cases and to direct them to nearest government hospital which is presumably better equipped to deal with paper-work formalities involved. Doctors normally prefer to block all pathways leading to medico-legal complications since they are as ignorant of laws as legalists are of medical invasions. For private practitioners, time brings them their earnings and all legal avenues are invariably time consuming. The more conscientious ones, in keeping with their moral duty, do provide minimum first aid and rush the patient to a government or a municipal hospital which is legally bound to accept all accident cases. The government hospitals maintain records of all such medico-legal cases so that even if disposal of a case is delayed, the doctor on duty, whoever he be, could produce records before the court. The cross-examination of the government doctor, who is not an eye-witness, then becomes a mere formality unlike in the case of private doctors who can be grilled in cross-examination.

Doctor as a Witness

Normally, those who have witnessed the accident are cited/ produced as witnesses. However, a doctor is ushered in to help a victim on the spot or later to treat the victim when shifted to a hospital. He invariably comes into the picture after an accident has occurred but still, in a court of law, his role is very significant for, on his deposition, the balance of justice tilts in favour of a complainant or an accused.

The doctor's assessment regarding injuries to an accident victim is of great importance not only for a victim but also for a person who may be charged, as is invariably done in vehicular accident cases, for having committed an offence by rash and negligent driving. Rashness and negligence are terms descriptive of the nature of an act which causes a particular harm. They do not describe the consequence or the nature of harm. In fact, if while driving a car nobody is injured or nobody dies, that does not *prima facie* mean that driving was neither rash nor negligent and, on the other hand, if ten people are injured or if some die in a road car accident that does not pre-suppose that a driver was rash or negligent. Therefore, rashness and negligence are the nature of the act which need to be correlated to the accident for purposes of prosecution (For details see chapter on 'medical negligence').

Having treated a victim, the doctor is required to render evidence as regards the injuries incurred, the condition of the patient and his assessment of whether the injuries could have been caused under the facts and circumstances as made out in the case either by the prosecution or the accused or yet again, for awarding compensation to the victim. Therefore, when a doctor is treating a patient involved in a road accident he should be particular to note down the site, extent and nature of injuries including dimensions of the wound with their clear description. He should treat a patient not only with the medical knowledge at his disposal but should go a step further to question the persons who have brought him from the site of accident, regarding the nature of accident and also record his opinion on the victims injuries *vis-a-vis* accident as this would be helpful later in medico-legal evidence of the case.

Every qualified specialist is expected to have undergone training in general medicine and surgery and is qualified to treat an accident case in an emergency or even otherwise. However, having provided emergency attention and evaluated the injury, it would be his duty to advise specialised intervention unless, in his opinion, no such specialised treatment was necessitated by facts of the case and condition of the patient. The doctor while treating a patient involved in an accident must bear in mind, at every point of time, that the line of treatment adopted can be a subject matter of litigation in a court of law. This word of caution is not intended to restrain a doctor from treating a patient in whichever manner he deems fit. All the same, a doctor might find himself cornered during cross-examination if being a gynaecologist he has treated or comes to give evidence in an orthopaedic case or being an ayurvedic doctor, has ventured into injecting antibiotics.

In practice, it is not uncommon for such and similar problems to arise. In an accident case, the victim who had suffered a colles' fracture,* was treated at a government hospital by an orthopaedic surgeon and the routine procedure of reduction under anaesthesia and plaster followed. A case was filed in the metropolitan magistrate's court. It took four to five years for the matter to reach the stage when the medical witness was summoned to depose. By that time, the orthopaedic surgeon who had treated the fracture had expired and on the date of the court hearing, another orthopaedic surgeon on duty either could not be spared or was reluctant to give his time to court proceedings. The doctor who was deputed by the hospital with the papers was a gynaecologist who was not much of an expert in orthopaedics and the prosecutor and the judge wanted to be enlightened as to what exactly was the case of the prosecution.

The defence lawyer, however, knew exactly that a colles' fracture could be caused by a fall on the outstretched hand and not by a direct vehicular impact. The gynaecologist naturally was caught in the net of intricacies and on further interrogation, his evidence proved to be of no aid to the prosecution.[201]

And such case studies can fill volumes.

Anyway, be that as it may. Doctors handling accident cases, which could be court cases at any point of time, must take extra care to have their records clear, including, the date of admission, the date of surgery and all the intervening procedures with clarity. There is no gainsaying that doctors are normally respected by courts and are simply expected to enlighten courts on medical condition and to answer questions to the best of their ability. It is not as if they are being examined on their knowledge of medical science. In reality, a clever lawyer cross-examining the doctor, invariably succeeds in imbalancing him/her to the advantage of the opponent.

Anyway, responsibility of the doctor is, firstly, to diagnose the problem; secondly, to understand the nature of accident and to form an opinion regarding the manner in which injury could have occurred, considering medical aspects of the case. Of utmost importance is the bearing of the doctor for, in a court, he represents the medical profession. To maintain dignity of the medical profession and reply with confidence while being in the box are keys to success. Let not a doctor become a tool in the hands of a lawyer. Lastly, doctors, specially those who come from government hospitals, it is felt, believe that they are acting as witnesses for the prosecution, namely the State, and therefore invariably, attempt to

---

[201] A case in the personal knowledge of the authoress.

depose against the accused whatever be the reality. Many a time, the explanations put forth by them tend to defy logic and commonsense. That is not to be expected from any doctor and his morals should make him place facts of the case and logic together before he enters a court of law as a medical witness.

Conclusion

In conclusion, a doctor as a significant personna of professional society has a great responsibility in the prevention of road accidents as also in the handling of accident victims as well as tendering legal evidence. The more their time and services are valued by the bureaucracy, the court, the legal men and the masses whom they seek to serve, the greater would be the benefit accruing to the suffering humanity and most of all the victims of accident whose sufferance is great and calls for immediate attention which none other than the medical man can give. And so can all serving segments combine to work for benefit of humanity.

AIDS and The Law

Auto Immune Deficiency Syndrome(AIDS), a multi-dimensional terrorising problem, requires an indepth study from many faceted prism, being medical and psychological, ethical and religious, social and humanitarian, economic and legal, *et al*, often overlapping and invariably interacting. AIDS, a disease, spreading rather like an epidemic, often emerges as a complex phenomenon, with all its consequential discriminatory disciplines, thus calling for societal literacy on the subject and constant intervention of laws.

Challenging confusion, medico-legal, socio-legal and ethico-legal problems concerning this dreaded and deadly disease, have been clouding the minds of intelligentsia, more so the scientists, ever since its first case, reported in 1981 from Los Angeles,[202] after which an estimated 1,00,000 adults have shown Human Immuno Virus deficiency (HIV) positive worldwide.[203] The following decade and a half have witnessed a human calamity, and medical naivete, requiring an urgent need for intensifying medical update, awareness, study, analytical dissection and above all an open dialogue. For example, impact of HIV in developing countries is multiplied by age-old curses of humankind, poverty and illiteracy, largely circumventing effectivity of health care schemes and health

---

[202]Prof S.R. Bhansali, "Need for law to control HIV/AIDS in India" 389 vol 2, Proceedings of Interdisciplinary International Conference on AIDS -Law and Humanity, The Indian Law Institute, New Delhi (1995).

[203]Tobi Saidel, Bill Rau, "Uses of HIV/AIDS Epidemologic Data, Estimates and Projections in Policy Development" 211, vol III, *id.*

education programmes, thereby reducing chances of containing spread of the disease in the community at large. In the meanwhile, while we prevaricate and indulge our complacency, global studies regularly shoot out with alarming clarity, statistics revealing rapidly rising toll of HIV infection, specially in developing countries, with India fast becoming the AIDS capital of Asia. The statistics are indeed a clarion call for concern. Health agencies like the World Health Organisation (WHO) and the Harvard AIDS Institute have estimated that India will have 2,000,000 to 5,000,000 AIDS infected patients by the end of the century.[204] Mumbai, according to Indian Health Organisation (IHO), is the country's AIDS capital.[205] An epidemiological study conducted by Tata Institute of Social Sciences places the number of HIV cases in Mumbai at 40,000.[206]

It is estimated that, globally, over 21 million are currently infected with HIV/AIDS, with ninety per cent of them in the developing world, and that nearly 8,500 people are being freshly infected with HIV everyday.[207] According to WHO, globally, eight to ten million people are estimated to be infected by this virus, a pathway to AIDS, of which about one-third are women.[208] The highest incidence of infection is found in 21 to 35 years age group.[209] Those who die are young, perhaps in their early twenties.

The worst dilemma, producing an aura of scare around the disease, is the knowledge that there is as yet no curative therapy or prophylactic vaccine for this infection,[210] or a vaccine that can prevent asymptomatic HIV infection from converting to AIDS, thus unrestrainedly spreading the epidemic. The best relief however is

---

[204]*The Statesman* (Delhi ed) 30 November 1996.
[205]*Sunday Observer* 18 August 1996.
[206]*Ibid.*
[207]*The Hindu* (Madras ed) 26 November 1996.
[208]Panos Dossier, *Triple Jeopardy : Women and AIDS* 1 (1990) Panos Publication Ltd.
[209]Rupa Chinai, *Times of India* (Bombay ed) 15 December 1995.
[210]"Policies, Laws and Regulations : Potential Barriers to HIV/AIDS Education and Services" 47, at 49, vol III, supra n 203.

the news that members of WHO are hopeful of an effective vaccine by end of the century. Intensive research to prolong survival of victims of AIDS, specially children, is now under way.

However, even hope of a possible vaccine and optimistic declaration of the possibility of development of some modes of containing the monster in the near future, are often diminished with factual data of global spread of the virus, which is surely encroaching much faster than results achieved by scientists for its prevention.

Whatever be chances of survival of humankind from this draconian disease in future, today it has to be borne in mind that on account of long latent period for transference of symptoms from HIV to fully developed AIDS, estimates of AIDS cases, as of today, at best touch an approximation. Therefore the subject of AIDS, as needs to be presently projected and sought to be tackled, has to be more from point of prevention rather than the cure.

AIDS - The Disease

AIDS, a communicable viral disease caused by HIV, has an inherent capacity to diminish, or rather destroy, the immunity mechanism of the body making an affected individual highly susceptible to infection. After surreptitiously entering the human body, the concerned virus, slowly and gradually, over a period of years, destroys defence mechanism resulting in a HIV affected system, subsequently developing into AIDS. Several asymptomatic years, often referred to as the latent period, may lapse before development of AIDS, posing crucial problems, as, during this period, seemingly healthy adults can unknowingly and unintentionally infect others. For example, a person may be a potential virus carrier or a dormant AIDS victim without being at all aware of it. If such a person unknowingly gets married, he may be in fact setting up an entire family of AIDS affected victims. HIV *per se* is not a killer infection but secondary infection and malignancy that occur in 'immuno compromised persons' are responsible for immense suffering that precedes death.

The common vehicle of transmission of HIV virus, which thrives in a nutritive medium and cannot survive outside the body, is through blood, seminal or vaginal fluid. It is generally transmitted *via* unprotected physical relation with an infected partner irrespective of the gender; *via* impure or infected blood transfusion and use of infected needles, syringes or surgical instruments or again *via* an infected mother to her progeny during pregnancy itself, or during a vertical transmission at birth.[211] AIDS, though transmittable, is not *per se* infectious and does not affect another through mere casual contact.[212]

At the same time, no detectable co-relation has been established between risk of transmission of the infection and the stage of the disease. Some may be most infective even in their asymptomatic phase just after getting contaminated by HIV, others exhibiting symptoms may not be infective at all. In other words, the development of symptoms and the infectivity of the disease do not seem to bear any correlation. This erratic nature of the disease can keep an affected person blissfully ignorant of his own plight, while posing a grave danger to his healthy partner. Also the disease lacks predictability to such an extent that in case of an HIV affected mother delivering twins it is quite possible for one twin to be infected while the other is normal and healthy.

Within this set of variables, if one has to extract a symptological uniformity, then the description could be as follows: a mild bout of illness may be caused by infection but a latent asymptomatic period which may even extend to about 10 years can follow. Even during this phase, laboratory investigations do indicate weakening of body's immune system, with oral thrush and

---

[211]See, Robert A Glick, Law, Ethics and HIV 19 (1993) UNDP Regional Project.
[212]*Id* at 391.

skin problems not being uncommon. In quite a few cases, this is then followed by, a phase of ailments like persistent cough, generalised pruritic dermatitis,* recurrent herpes zoster,* oropharyngeal candidasis* and generalised lymphadenopathy*.[213] In the case of women, early manifestations of HIV infection may include, in addition to the above mentioned symptoms, persistent gynaecological complaints.[214]

The more serious symptoms include night sweats, weight loss and diarrhoea or major illnesses such as prolonged fever, severe form of pneumonia* , pneumocystic carinii* (PCP) or an aggressive tumor, Kaposi's sarcoma* (KS), various other infections which attack several organs including the nervous system. This is the most critical stage of an AIDS victim.

AIDS - And Women

The glaring global statistics depicting that more and more women are being infected by the virus, and that, her unborn child is vulnerable to catching the disease during pre-natal phase itself, and is doomed to death within the first five years of his existence, has drawn the concern of scientists and social organisations the world over to correlation of AIDS with women.

These stark realities combined with the fact that at present, while constituting seventy per cent of the world's 1.3 billion poorest citizens, women are required to shoulder two-thirds of world's working hours, while earning only one-tenth of the world's income,[215] thus evidencing harsh economic realities and a high

---

*See Glossary.

[213]See, Dr D Sengupta, "AIDS - Diagnosis and Control", 283 *Swasth Hind* (Nov -Dec 1990).

[214]A. Willoughby, "Clinical Science and Trials," rapporteur session, *Abstracts of VIth International Conference on AIDS*, San Francisco, June 1990: See, supra n 208.

[215]Cheryl G Healton, M Lyndon Haviland & Ram Kairam, "Challenges of AIDS Prevention for Women in Both the Developing and Developed World" 325, vol 2, *supra* n 202.

degree of poverty, or rather their limited economic power, resulting in the pattern of rural to urban migration coupled with family instabilities, low educational attainment and cultural barriers, often combining to make AIDS prevention for women a challenge.

The WHO substantiates the victimology of women with AIDS declaring eight million women, worldwide, to have been already infected with HIV, and, by the year 2000, an estimate that, sixteen million women would have been infected with a death toll of over 4 million.[216] The menace could be curbed by compulsory screening of women for HIV during pregnancy. This suggestion has many advocates despite the fact that intra-uterine infection cannot be prevented even with therapeutic intervention but, counselling for termination of pregnancy in early stages could be helpful in containing the disease in children. Termination of pregnancy, though medically advised, may not be palatable to would be parents, on emotional grounds in which case they cannot be compelled, but still there would be many who would agree to termination in the interest of the family. The more difficult cases will be those whose religion prohibits them from so doing.[217] However, detailing dire consequences and dangers involved, may, sooner or later, strike their inner chord making them more susceptible to the idea of abortion.

Irrespective of HIV, pregnancy *per se* weakens immune system of a woman increasing her vulnerability to numerous infections. If a woman is in addition a HIV positive victim, her defence mechanism would be at a low ebb making her more prone to treacherous complications. Moreover, well established is the fact that maternal HIV infection oft-times leads to pre-mature delivery and intra-uterine growth retardation, exposing her to double jeopardy, of having to deal with her own malady as well as grave

[216]*Id* at 326.
[217]*Ibid.*

responsibility of an infected progeny.

With this dismal picture, fate of an unborn has today become a major concern of pre-natal management, gravity of the problem enhanced due to weak immune system in infancy, resulting in rapid progression of HIV infection and pediatric AIDS with quick fatal culmination.

A baby whose mother is HIV positive can be infected in three ways: pre-natally (HIV has been detected in very early foetuses and in blood of the umbilical cord); during delivery by mother's infected blood or vaginal secretions; or, in a very few documented cases, also from mother's milk.[218]

Yet, in majority of cases, due to the latent period of development from HIV to AIDS, infection must have had its first seed sown during teens. The spread of AIDS in women has been found to be relatively slower. Even so, bearing in mind latent period for development of disease from HIV positive to full blown AIDS estimates of AIDS cases can at best touch an approximation.

WHO predicts that 5-10 million HIV infected children will have been born by the year 2000.[219] Their death trap would grab them before they have a chance to bloom. The unaffected 75% are likely to be orphaned before they reach five years of age and would have to face consequential harsh realities.

The fate of an AIDS affected girl child is still more heart-wrenching; her calamitous condition being, in turn, intimately correlated to her mother suffering from AIDS from whom it is transmitted. Let's take an example: a girl child dies before her fifth birthday for her only crime that she is born of a father infected with

---

[218]S. Blanche and others, "A prospective study of infants born to women seropositive for HIV", *New England Journal of Medicine*, 1643-8, no 25 vol 320 (22 June 1989), See *Supra* n 208, at 43.

[219]See, 45th World Health Assembly, Provisional Agenda Item 33, WHA 45, 35 (14th May, 1992).

HIV from a contaminated needle. He in turn, though unknowingly, had passed on the infection to his wife. The little child was born AIDS-infected, disease transmitted to her by her mother, who in turn acquired it from a diseased husband.

An indepth study of the impact of AIDS on women entering the institution of matrimony brings to light their pathetic fate, as distinct from vulnerability of a single woman. A few case studies of healthy women caught in the web of disease following matrimony, bring out some heart wrenching realities.

Consider this situation: a young girl with all bright dreams of a rosy future enters into a marriage bond confident that heavens will be hers till 'death do us part.' Possibility A: she is in blissful ignorance of affliction of her husband already tested HIV positive but which fact has been skilfully concealed. In the natural course of events gleefully, she bears her first child. The virus has, in the meanwhile, done its job and she has already been 'blessed' with the virus by him. Latent period for HIV to progress to AIDS for a child being relatively small, the child is doomed to develop AIDS within first four years and then to die.

The young girl who has borne her first little one lives to see the death of her first born. By now she learns about HIV infection that took away her treasure and knows that she cannot ever risk having a child again. Question arises: how should law extend its hands to her since, in reality, it is the husband who has, knowingly and fraudulently, and by concealing his affliction before or after marriage infected her? No divorce can compensate or offer a solution to the problem of this young girl as she has not only got diseased for life, but has lost all hopes of a normal future and of ever being a mother, a just desire of every woman who enters portals of matrimony.

Should the husband not be criminally prosecuted for having committed such a fraud in marriage? Or, on the other hand, should he be allowed to go scot free on mercy grounds of already being a victim of the draconian disease and his rapidly approaching death? In any case, would criminal prosecution of the man or even a liberal compensation be an answer to suffering caused to the victim?

In case compassion is the answer, is it not a licence to committing crime against the innocent partner, time and again? What would be the deterrent to other similar men from ruining the lives of young innocent victims at the very threshold of their bloom?

Possibility B: suppose in the above case, the husband, having nurtured the HIV virus for quite a few years prior to the marriage and now suffering from full blown AIDS, dies. The young girl would acquire the status of widowhood with all the accompanying pangs, before ever having had the chance to bloom. Nor can she expect a sympathetic treatment or security from her insensitive in-laws for whom she is now an outcast and a burdensome mouth to feed. If in the meanwhile, rejected by her in-laws and parents alike, she has already caught the disease, who is going to look after her for the rest of her diseased life? Does the law and the State hold any hope for help or solace or solution for her?

Possibility C: the husband suffers from HIV infection of which he was not aware. The couple lead a normal life for some time till the knowledge dawns on them both and perhaps that of the immediate relatives. More often than not, the in-laws would blame her for ruining the life of their son. It is not impossible that even the husband will turn around and blame her for his misery. Depression and gloom cast their shadow not only on the couple but two households who have come together in a common bondage. Looming large is the prospect of becoming a young infected widow ; but what is her solution?

Firstly, being unable to conform to traditional societal norms, she is regarded as a social failure. Secondly, with the woman constantly avoiding company, life becomes more burdensome with her becoming reticent and introvert. Her sick and diseased condition infuses her with a feeling of being unwanted, she lacks security, the basic requirement of every human being. Her psychological condition is compounded by her inability to find employment and thereby sustainance for herself. Under these circumstances, she becomes a social apparition and an economic burden. In case she does find herself an employment, she has to live under constant trauma of concealing her true condition for fear of being shunned by her associates, for once it is known she is HIV positive, in all probability, not only will she lose her job but even her reputation. Society would raise its ugly head to adopt an attitude of social boycott against her.

Even the most extreme of extremist male chauvinists would agree that a better answer would be to aim at preventing such doomed unions rather than live with dumb and deaf laws which offer no viable solution. To prohibit and prevent marriages doomed from their very inception would be one of the greatest services that legislators could render to society. A glaringly obvious solution is to make registration of marriages compulsory and a health check up for HIV status immediately prior to the marriage an essential requirement.

Realising the unsurmountable difficulties faced by an AIDS affected woman, the Beijing Platform for Action, in their effort to control spread of the disease, explained that:

"Women, who represent half of all adults newly infected with HIV/AIDS and other sexually transmitted diseases, have emphasised that social vulnerability and the unequal power relationships between women and men are obstacles to safe sex,..... The consequences of HIV/AIDS reach beyond women's health to their role as mothers and caregivers and their contribution to the economic support of their families. The social, developmental and health consequences of HIV/AIDS and other sexually transmitted diseases need to be seen from a gender perspective."[220]

Under these circumstances, a hectic propaganda to bring about awareness of magnitude of the problem is essential for realisation to dawn on the world that hard core methodologies aiming at attacking the root cause of he problem have to be listed and tackled firmly with an iron hand.

AIDS - And Law

In this era of jet-speed scientific advancement in medical field, with "health for all by 2000 A.D." as the avowed government policy, an alarming spread of AIDS has hardly drawn active concern, although not as much that it deserves. In a confused scenario of increasing complexities, law and medicine, two holy implements of service to humanity, have to join their forces as solution finding faculties and the laws must at all times move forward to meet the necessities of times. Continuous systematic changes in relevant laws in the form of deletions, alterations and/or additions, must necessarily cope with volcanic changes of a fast developing social environment, including health hazards.

As it stands today, the dilemma of ever-rising cases of AIDS has baffled physicians the world over and enmeshed them in a web of medical research, engulfing them with problems never encountered before. The legal giants are caught in the problem of legalising enforced protection to healthy humans to save them from disease and destruction. The medical scientists may succeed in discovering curative therapy, but the legal minds have to engineer appropriate workable instruments to combat social danger of spread of AIDS by regulating human behaviour.

---

[220]Paragraph 99, Platform for Action adopted by the United Nations Fourth World Conference on Women: Equality, Development and Peace, Beijing, China, Advance Unedited Draft, (15 September 1995), in D C Jayasuriya (ed), *HIV Law And Humans Rights - Text and Materials* 244 (1995) (UNDP Regional Project on HIV and Development).

On 18 August 1989, in a bid to fulfil or at least initiate a move towards the objective, 'The Acquired Immuno Deficiency Syndrome (AIDS) Prevention Bill' was introduced in *Rajya Sabha*,[221] to control the liberty of private citizens, giving sweeping powers to health authorities and government. The Bill proposed to clothe health authorities with powers to subject prostitutes and their customers to compulsory testing and also to prohibit professional blood donors from donating blood or any organ. While not providing for compulsory AIDS test for foreign students or other foreigners coming to India, this Bill sought to compel a professional blood donor, or one who gives his blood more than once within a period of three months for monetary consideration, to get his blood tested for the presence of HIV antibodies in his blood, every time, prior to donation, and required him to donate only if such test proved that he was clear from HIV antibodies. However, this Bill has not yet seen the light of the day.

Suffice it to say that some strict measures need to be urgently devised and introduced on a war footing if Indian masses are to be protected from death and destruction by this draconian disease. In the arena of matrimonial laws, specific provisions suggested on priority basis are:

- registration of marriage to be made compulsory and subject to medical fitness certificate, including absence of HIV, in all cases;
- well equipped laboratories, run by government or other authorised doctors and/or government hospitals should alone be licenced to give medical fitness certificate;
- in case of false certification, including cases of HIV infection, severe punishment should be meted out expeditiously to the culprit doctor / technician;
- provisions should be propagated through radio, TV, and other

[221]Bill No : XX of 1989, introduced in the Upper House of Parliament.

advanced communication technology in order to reach out information regarding legislation to every nook and corner of India where illiteracy, ignorance and poverty abound.

Such and many more provisions are worth at least an open dialogue. We cannot forget that the laxity and absence of sanctions and the pathological delays, ingrained in Indian judicial system, are harming human life and society and need to be overhauled as an essential gesture of compassion to innocents who are being infected everyday.

Of course, compulsory registration of marriage should in any case be introduced, for it has a clear cut advantage of establishing the relationship of husband and wife without any unnecessary hassles now required to be gone through specially in matters involving matrimonial crimes.[222] As of today, a number of cases are pending before the judiciary only for evidence of a legally contracted valid marriage.

Some further crucial policy decisions on this issue which need urgent application of mind are:

- considering the inevitable risk of transmission of HIV by an infected partner to a healthy spouse and inability of a normal physical relation without incurring grave danger of transmission of the infection to future offspring of the union, sanctions against HIV positive to enter into a matrimonial alliance, need to be introduced;
- if a person suffering from AIDS or AIDS-Related-Diseases (ARD) or even asymptomatic HIV infection, knowingly enters into a matrimonial tie without disclosing affliction to the proposed spouse, concealment be recognised as a crime, a matrimonial fraud;

[222]Poornima Advani, Crime in Marriages : A Broad Spectrum 74 (1995) Gopushi Publishers, Mumbai.

- law must provide heavy compensation for such victims of fraud;
- knowing high incidence of pre-natal transmission and the fact that, in all probability, a child born to an AIDS affected mother will also carry the infection and be doomed to death before he can bloom, there being no effective medication so far, an expectant woman must compulsorily be made to undergo abortion, for in case a child is born, more often than not, he will have to grow up as an orphan and the management of life of an AIDS affected orphan child with compound psychological insecurity, would be, to say the least, a most devastating responsibility. An incidental question arises as to who should bear the brunt of such a responsibility?
- should a non-affording or abandoned AIDS victim be kept alive by indefinite medication on state expense?

Conclusion

It stands to reason that with no immediate prospect of a widely available vaccine or cure for HIV, the key to controlling AIDS lies in regulating human behaviour. No doubt, basic rights of an AIDS victim in the form of right to life, right to live with human dignity, right to employment and a whole gamut of human rights need attention, however, with statistics being thrown in our faces by the WHO and danger signals ticking away menacingly, even more essential is to introduce strictest disciplines to contain disease and prevent fresh inputs. After all prevention is better than cure and if the licentiate ways of living and entertaining have brought AIDS to India as a national calamity, apart from rigorous domestic education and sealing vulnerable borders of the nation more effectively to illegal immigrants, the whole lot of tourists from under developed and developing countries who visit the country throughout the year to enjoy laxities prohibited in their own countries but freely available in India and, in the bargain, infect the kidnapped and needy minors, recklessly made to trade in known areas, need to be checked for HIV positive at all the entry points as a pre-condition for crossing the barriers. Such and many more such measures surely need to be introduced on a war footing to save the nation from utter doom.

It cannot be gainsaid that carving a pathway to the solution of these problems would definitely require active concern and concerted efforts of legal experts who have until now been grappling within cobwebs of legal *versus* ethical requirements. Even when faced with human disasters, law-givers shy away under fear that they may be invading the socio-ethico-medico-legal fields. The role of mass literacy and social awareness cannot be over emphasised. In fact, when in India a positive step was taken by a marriage bureau to find partners for HIV-positive victims and advertisements in this regard appeared in the press, eight prospective brides responded and all of them thought "HIV positive" was an educational qualification. However, time has come for all faculties to stop prevaricating, come together on a common platform and respond to the clarion call of the statistics to awake, arise, act and save humanity from pain, suffering and doom, for the alarming spread of the disease is indeed leading to a pathetic situation.[223]

If we perform our duty to humankind with determination, dedication and devotion, we need not lose heart. We, the professionals, can still save the nation.

[223]"India has the largest number of HIV infected perople in the world. There is increased trafficking of women and children in India. The country is also witnessing a rising trend of HIV infected women. It appears that HIV is fast percolating from the high risk group to the general population and from urban to rural areas, *Times of India* (Mumbai ed) 2 December 1997.

Euthanasia-The Eternal Enigma

Mercy killing, an enigma facing society the world over, is one of those subjects of human concern which despite an endless debate, has not and probably will not yield an unanimous decision. To permit or not to permit? The taking away of a human life, should it at all be even open to discussion? Yet, however unsurmountable a proposition, a constant tussle has been raging for years on end in different corners of the world between schools with varied opinions.

In the past, under early Greek[224] and Roman[225] laws, a man's life and liberty and the life and liberty of his wife, children and slaves were considered to be his personal property, to be disposed off at his whims and fancies, even by bartering them away for pecuniary gains. The right of every man to consent to any injury being caused to him or his dependents, in its widest possible connotation, extended to the right to take away life of his dependants or himself and, as a corollary, to refuse medical treatment at any stage. Therefore, the question of permissibility of euthanasia did not arise, rather was considered an off-shoot of the then prevalent conditions. Mercy killing was acceptable and so was suicide. No civil or criminal liability could ensue in consequence of anything done with the person's 'consent'; the term thus played an aggressive role in the law of torts and the criminal jurisprudence of the past.

---

[224]Supra n 44.
[225]Supra n 45.

With development of the concept of society, old notions changed and human life was brought within the protective wings of the State. It was thence the primary duty of the State, and a responsible citizen as part of the State, to preserve and conserve human life, thus eliminating all control of an individual over his own life, his wife's life no longer his to barter. However, with State taking over this right, a parallel duty, of protecting life of individuals was cast on it which it performed through an elaborate police force and other security measures. From then on, it was only the State which had a right to terminate life, capital punishment being permitted in various countries including India. This was the state of affairs as existed in those early times and in which we survive even today.

Under these circumstances, no person has a right to take away his own life or permit or direct any other person to take it away. Hence attempted suicide1[226] and mercy killing[227] continue to be punishable under the penal laws of India.

Of late, some countries have legalised euthanasia, *albeit,* with selective precautionary measures and others have begun to consider the issue seriously. Australia's Northern Territory Right of the Terminally Ill Act, the world's first legislation authorising euthanasia (1 July 1996),[228] requires that two doctors must confirm that a patient is terminally ill, suffering unbearable pain, while a psychiatrist is required to affirm that the patient is not suffering from a treatable clinical depression. The patient is still required to wait for seven days before signing necessary papers and another 48 hours before life is terminated by a lethal drug.

Euthanasia

'Euthanasia', literally means an easy and painless death, hope

[226]S. 309, Indian Penal Code 1860: see Appendix A-Part B.
[227]S. 300 Exception 5, *id.*
[228]*The Pioneer* (Delhi ed) 5 October 1996.

and just desire of every human being. In its liberalised interpretation, it means 'mercy killing' or, the voluntary termination of life of someone suffering from an incurable disease, mental or physical, or from an irreparable effect of serious injury; or killing or aiding to extinguish life of a person on his own request or otherwise, whether with or without his consent.

Every human being inherently dreads death. Man by basic instinct is endowed with a desire for self-preservation,[229] the spark of life being the main flame of human existence, endeavour and enterprise. A person who sincerely desires and pleads for an end to existence, casting to winds his intense instinct to live, must be naturally moved by deep rooted unbearable mental torture and physical suffering, making his very breath a painful burden. It is only when the intensity of suffering reaches beyond the capacity of human endurance, that a thought to extinguish life transforms itself into an urge to die and that too in rare cases.

Enigma of mercy killing invariably revolves around victims of suffering. On the one hand, lie the uncared for aged and critically ill, both categories doomed to a miserable meaningless existence till end of their life, and on the other, the genetically defective born or unborn children, afflicted, from inception, with either physical deformities or mental disabilities or both. The child so born, or still worse, afflicted in infancy, is doomed to become a life-time burden, a mental trauma, an economic tragedy and a social stigma on parents, home and society, to say nothing of life itself.

Entire debate concerning euthanasia pivots around the ethico-logical reasoning that favours ending the endless misery of suffering souls by terminating their life, or may be just suspending aids that keep the light burning, but fear that any legislation sanctioning euthanasia must carry with it the dangers of misuse, keeps the step untrodden.

---

[229]Supra n 123, at 126.

A few critical cases, living either a tragic existence or a vegetative life, are herein reiterated with a view to aid deliberations whether, ethically and/or legally, flames within such lives should be kept burning or compassionately allowed to extinguish. Would the first option be compassion and the second a murder, or would the first one be irrational cruelty and second liberation?

Tragic Realities

The two well known and reported tales of Aruna Shanbag and Gangadhar are worth being reiterated.[230] Aruna, a young nurse, was raped in the nurses room at the Cardio Thoracic Centre, King Edward Memorial Hospital, Mumbai, on 27 November 1973. Violence had accompanied the rape. More specifically, a dog chain was wound tightly around her neck by a criminal rapist, resulting in diminished oxygen supply to her brain, thus making her lapse into a stage of coma in which she lingers till today. Even in her present state, her subconscious mind revolts against any male voice.

"She responds to friendly voices but never to a male voice. If she hears a male voice she shrieks and shrinks away".[231]

Aruna is doomed for the rest of her life to a state of utter helplessness - a once useful blossoming life utterly wasted. For two decades and odd years, the flame of life has been burning, she an object of compassion, yet a life not worth living, for all her near and dear ones have forsaken her and she continues to breathe in the hospital wherein her life became a tragedy.

The other soul stirring case is of Gangadhar[232] who, during an epileptic fit, tumbled face downward into blazing firewood. The face, mutilated by flames and horrible to a human eye, was sought to be treated by plastic surgeons of K.E.M. Hospital with twenty-

---

[230]Personal case study by the authoress. See Poornima Advani, "Euthanasia : the Eternal Enigma", *The Afternoon Despatch & Courier* 9 (Bombay ed) 30 April 1993.
[231]*Ibid.*
[232]*Ibid.*

three cosmetic surgeries performed on him over a period of ten years.

The difference in these two cases basically is that whereas Aruna's brain is permanently damaged leaving her selectively oblivious to the environment surrounding her, Gangadhar continues to survive with a normal brain, face still miserably mutilated, a horror to the beholders, his own looks constantly reminding him and making him conscious of the tragedy in his life.

Yet another tragic story is that of little Aayush, a victim of an incurable heart disease, which is as touching.[233]

"I experienced all the pain, despair and anguish that I had to when Aayush was suffering... Miracles don't happen and it is better to face reality. I was relieved when he passed away. He was no longer in pain. ...Just watching him suffer would make me sick... Aayush was totally bedridden and what he went through was sheer torture...I kept praying and pleading with the doctor's to let him go."[234]

Despite this anguish, doctors continued their efforts to keep the flame of life burning but the pre-determined end creeped in. Pathetic category of cases like Aruna touch the very core of human heart and ring bells of compassion with a clarion call: should human agency, whether individually or as a panel collectively, be given the right to put an end to existing life or should no man have a right to blow off the spark of life since, no doubt, it is not given to man to create it? The question has to be answered or rather debated while hearing a pathetic cry for mercy killing by Aayush's own mother which depicts an otherwise horrifying end that an incurable painful disease could lead to.

Equally debatable is the case of terminally ill patients suffering beyond human capacity and without an iota of hope for survival,

---

233 *Savvy* (Bombay ed) October 1995.
234 *Ibid.*

longing for an end to their lives, the only solution to their indescribable suffering. One such example is of Ben Dent,[235] a 66 year old cancer patient who died at Darwin, Australia, aided by a computerised death machine called 'deliverance.' His note said, "the Church and State must remain seperate. If you disagree with voluntary euthanasia, then don't use it, but please don't deny me the right to use it if and when I want to. For months I have been on a rollercoaster of pain made worse by the unwanted side-effects of painkillers."

While such tragedies can occur in the life span of any human being, there is another heart wrenching reality presented in birth of a defective child. The eternal question arises and continues to persist: whose life is it anyway and who should bear the burden of tending with care such a life? In fact, should such a life be tended to with compassion, care and caution or just be allowed to ebb away? In the latter case who should be the one to decide?

Fact or Fiction

To study the topic of 'mercy killing' from the dimension of the new born babes, a field study was undertaken by the authoress in the paediatric unit of K.E.M. Hospital, Mumbai, and many unusual, though true to life, thought provoking stories were revealed.

Around January 1993, a young male child weighing just about 700 grams was found outside Prabhadevi, Mumbai, by a police woman on duty. The child measured upto size of the palm of a human hand. This little one was abandoned, hidden totally in a sack which lay on the roadside and on inspecting the bag and laying her hands on its unusual contents, the woman rushed the babe to KEM Hospital. Head of Department of Neonatology, a very dedicated pediatrician, recalled with a look of concern writ large on her compassionate face: "we all thought at the intensive care

---

[235] *The Pioneer* (Delhi ed) 5 October 1996.

unit that this little one could not survive. The skin was not to be found, the child was bleeding all over because of fragile capillaries and suffered from pyogenic meningitis and pneumonia." This child could not suffer a human touch for the first one month as even minimal handling would cause severe bleeding. He was kept on intravenous diet of expensive proteins and aminoacids and feeding continued for two and a half months. At the age of three months, the child weighed 1.3 kilos, could be fed with a spoon, cried when hungry, responded to cuddling and was fondly named 'Shashi' by the staff of the hospital.[236]

Three small children born around the same time as Shashi and initially thought to be 'still born' were revived and kept in an intensive care unit on expensive medication in the pediatric unit. One of these, a child named Shobha, had suffered from the dangerous 'Salmonella infection' when she was just four days old but managed to survive. Shashi and Shobha were often together in the same ward. Whereas at the age of three months, Shashi made a tragic picture, Shobha looked near normal. It was a common sight at the ward to see mothers of sick babies envying Shobha and sympathising with Shashi.

Several questions continued to haunt the minds of all concerned: would Shashi be a normal child even if he lived? In any case, if this child did survive, who would shoulder the responsibility of a forsaken and possibly handicapped child? What would life and society have to offer him? In the circumstances in which he had been abandoned, it was only right to presume that life will really have nothing to offer him; still, did we have the right to do away with intensive medication and allow life to ebb away?

Till that stage doctors were keeping their fingers crossed as

---

[236]Case study by the author conducted in the neonatal ward of KEM Hospital, Mumbai. See also *supra* n 230.

until the baby had completed fourteen weeks it was difficult to determine whether neurologically he would grow up to be a normal child. In any case, whatever be his physical condition, he would definitely be an addition to the already overwhelming population of orphaned and abandoned children of the nation. If one may throw a wild guess, this child was surely an unwanted product of a free licentiate society, abandoned by the natural mother and may be not even having a known genetic father. The subject of mercy killing was often discussed, *albeit,* in hushed under-tones, while projecting into the future of this innocent babe.

However, human beings are almost always ignorant of the plans of destiny. The Master Planner's ways are inscrutable and unpredictable. So it was with this child. Shashi has today not only survived but is adopted by a loving Scottish couple. He is a normal child, although initially with delayed milestones, a child who plays with other children of peers in the Scottish school, living a perfectly normal life. On the other hand, Shobha has grown up in depressing surroundings primarily because her mother, stricken with poverty and accursed with an alcoholic husband has borne severe domestic violence and the child has throughout lacked loving upbringing that could have made her develop normally and bloom in security.

Another shocking true story is of a little one born with a huge tumor (cyclops) on the forehead, normal face divided into three parts by two deep and long fissures across the face. Every system above the neck was malfunctioning and every system below the neck was normal. The heart beat properly and lungs functioned normally. His birth was by a Cesarean section. This was the first delivery of the mother. Seeing the horrifying face of this babe, the father prevented hospital authorities from showing the child to the mother, his scare being that if his wife saw such an abnormal child she would never again agree to mother another one. The little baby was of no consequence to the father and he hurriedly donated the body for use in the anatomy museum. However, until alive, the hospital authorities had to discharge their duty. Neurosurgeons determined that not much of brain matter existed; plastic surgeons put their hands up; pediatric unit kept him alive in a separate room, on expensive drugs, but the child died within twenty-one days.[237] In any case, factually, it was known at birth that the child would be abnormal, a horrifying spectacle and an unwanted babe.

Yet, did doctors have a duty to preserve life till he did breathe? And even presuming they did have such a duty and performed it with all ingenuity at their command, who could predict whether the little one would live or die? And again, was it at all necessary to put in best effort available for an apparently unwanted, miserable life, even presuming it could be saved?

Such cases and many more bring us to importance of defining death to determine when such a life can be terminated. The Dutch Paediatric Association has also lobbied the government to allow euthanasia of infants when their expected quality of life was deemed too low.[238] In one case, which caused international outrage, life of a two day old Down's Syndrome baby with a correctable stomach problem was terminated.[239]

Death

Death has been described as an eventuality where medicine, law, ethics and religion hover around a human life during last moments of his existence in this world or rather in brief moments of his onward journey to the unknown world beyond. Being intrigued for want of a conclusive definition, scientists, world over, have been perpetually boggled with the question: what is death? Importance of this question has enhanced tenfold with advancement of technological innovations in science which have helped prolong life in a patient who would have, in the past, been 'deemed dead.'

---

[237] *Supra* n 230.
[238] *The Independent* (Bombay ed) 13 February 1993.
[239] *Ibid.*

Today, a physician is often faced with a situation where despite stoppage of normal breathing, patient is not dead and, even survives with help of artificial respiration; should such a patient be declared 'dead'? In medical world of today, absence of beating of the pulse, considered in days gone by as the criteria to determine death, is no longer a conclusive evidence.

Enigmas arising as a corollary to scientific innovations had set the medical professionals thinking long ago and in 1968, an Ad Hoc Committee of the Harvard Medical School set out to examine state of 'death' and came out with idea of existence of 'brain death' in a report entitled 'A Definition of Irreversible Coma.'[240]

It has been established that once a brain cell is damaged for more than a duration of three minutes, due to any cause, be it infection, lack of oxygen or insufficiency of glucose, it will never recover. On the contrary, these conditions have been cause of permanent handicap in immense number of children, ruined lives being kept alive only with aid of expensive life saving therapies, thus keeping sub-normal defective human beings alive. Many abnormal children born today, who would have normally passed into oblivion, being declared dead within minutes earlier, continue to breathe on artificial respirators, expensive drugs, innovative therapies and advanced technology. In some cases, near and dear ones, specially the prisoners of religious dictas, have to bear prolonged mental trauma, and economic disasters by the time the child is officially declared dead. Many parents overcome these aberrations, and, finding themselves unable to cope with expenses, even request that extra-ordinary measures taken to sustain life of the child born with abnormalities, nature-made or doctor-induced, be stopped but then doctor's duty of sustaining life as long as possible stands in the way. Thus do calamitous conditions and traumatic experiences continue.

---

[240]*Supra* n 150.

An ethical debate has been raging since long, in medico-legal fields, whether request to put an end to artificially aided existence of a suffering victim should be honoured and, if so, who should shoulder the burden of taking this horrendous step of literally withdrawing aids, thus allowing life to ebb out. If such a contingency does crop up, who should take the final decision: parents, physician, parents and physicians together; an ethics committee, legislature, courts or should the decision be left to God, the Creator of all?

Towards Legalising Mercy Killing

The backlash of penalising an attempt to commit suicide and mercy killing was primarily based on the premise that human life belonged to the State and an individual had no right to take away what did not belong to him. Hence, 'suicide' (killing one's own self), 'homicide' (killing another person) and even 'euthanasia' (mercy killing) had all fallen under the sword of penal laws.

In India, on 16 April 1994, a division bench of Supreme Court adjudged that a person had a right to take away his own life and punishment for attempt to commit suicide was 'cruel and irrational,' being violative of constitutional rights of a person.[241] The change in the think-tank of the judiciary raised various questions: did concept of 'humanisation' not take away unstinted monopoly of ownership of State over human life, *albeit* partially? If necessity of 'humanisation of laws' had prompted the Apex Court to attune 'this part of our criminal law to global wavelength',[242] by declaring provisions as unconstitutional, would not the next stage of 'global thinking' also prompt court to legalise mercy killing? Obviously, if suicide could be triggered by a complex and varied set of causes, euthanasia could probably be considered on *par*. However, while mentioning that "though it may be said that if suicide is held

---

[241] *Supra* n 177.
[242] *Id* at 429.

to be legal, the persons pleading for legal acceptance of passive euthanasia would have a winning point,"[243] they restricted scope of judgment to persons committing suicide.

It was being argued that euthanasia was akin to suicide as it was a voluntary request for aid to die. If right to die is recognised, why not right to take aid for dying from another? A natural corollary would be: should not a third person, a well-wisher, have the right to be a decision-making individual? Or, if not an individual, should not a body of persons be empowered to take this crucial decision?

However, before such controversial debates could make any appreciable headway, a constitutional bench of Supreme Court reviewed and reversed its earlier verdict,[244] declaring that provision of the Indian Penal Code which punishes attempt to commit suicide is not unconstitutional. It was observed that "the debate on the desirability of retaining such a penal provision of punishing attempted suicide,... are not sufficient to indicate that the provision is unconstitutional being violative of Article 14."[245]

Admittedly, a lot of thought energy would have to flow from the legal think-tank if, even in principle, mercy killing is sought to be legalised.

Ethical Viewpoint

Moralists and humanists take exception to mercy killing on numerous grounds: they stress that all life is revered as divinely ordained, created by Supreme Architect, man does not have a right to take away something which he cannot create or restore and that taking away life of a human being militates against human conscience. An argument is put forth that mercy killing is an irrevocable act and human fallacy being what it is, if later the

---

[243] *Id* at 427.

[244] *Smt. Gian Kaur v State of Punjab and others,* 1996 Cri.L.J. 1660 (SC).

[245] *Id* at 1667.

decision is discovered to be wrong, mistake done is final and non-rectifiable as an innocent ignorant consenting victim is put beyond power of humans to revive. The flame of life once put out cannot be rekindled.

The counter-thinkers argue that with rapid advancement in medical science, leading to miraculous inroads into nature, divinity and nature have to a certain extent been relegated as dictators of the past, being no more in exclusive control of human destinies. The grant of gift of motherhood to many a frustrated woman who, in recent past, had to live and die without progeny of their own, by artificial insemination and surrogacy, are but proofs of supremacy of science over nature.

Surely there can be no dispute to the boon that medical science has provided to humankind. However, quality of life even in a vegetative state, rather than its elongation, or creation artifically, is what is more significant in the debate and consideration of suject of euthanasia.

Spiritualistic Viewpoint

Arthur Ford speaking to Ruth Montegomery from the spirit world says: "No person has a right to take the life within himself, any more than that of another person, since all are a part of the Godhead..."[246] Thus, every soul, when he is to be born into this world, selects the pattern of life of each *janma* after reference to the heavenly computer, *akashic* records, and plans paying back of his past *karmas* during each life. Sickness and suffering are fastest prescriptions of paying back *karmic* debts. Who can have a right to question an individual's selection and/or tamper with what he has chosen to repay in this life? In any case, moralists, who give importance to sustaining life, do not shudder at quality of existence, suffering therefrom, coolly placing forth the theory of *karma* as a

[246]Ruth Montgomery, A *World Beyond* 41 (Fawcett Publication, Inc., Greenwich, Conn).

pacifying factor; that sickness and suffering being quickest ways of redeeming debit balances of bad actions of earlier births, whatever we may do, *karmas* have to be recompensated in this birth or next or still thereafter. Therefore, shirking punishment ordained by divinity would not serve a concrete purpose.

The spiritualistic approach goes on: life is sacred and therefore we must not extinguish spark of life even if the patient is in unbearable pain and suffocating suffering. The Judaeo-Christian faith considers euthanasia unacceptable; each human life is believed to be God's gift and thus putting someone to death is a sin; thou shalt not kill.[247]

The counter thinking runs: if life is sacred why do we kill other creations? Why do humans eat sheep and goat, fish, fowl and frogs? Why does law prescribe capital punishment for even human beings? Why does law exonerate a man to kill another in exercise of his right to self defence? And if all these are daily occurrences of life, then why not permit ending a painful existence?

The debate goes on and on.

Legal Viewpoint

Mercy killing, under S. 300 Excep 5 of Indian Penal Code, has been classified as culpable homicide not amounting to murder, in case death is of a person above age of 18 years, and prescribed punishment runs to imprisonment for a maximum period of 10 years;[248] death of a person below 18, howsoever merciful, would still amount to murder. Moreover, grant of the right to consent does not extend beyond the suffering party himself. Offence of murder is merely brought on par with homicide but the criminal liability prevails.

Primarily, self-preservation is a basic instinct of man. However,

[247]The Holy Bible, Exodus 20: The Ten Commandments.
[248]*Supra* n 227.

extreme stress and strain do create an emotional imbalance, at times, instigating man to contemplate ending his own life. Even such situations are often accompanied by inner conflict and fiery debate on a choice between life and death in the person's own mind making him confused worse confounded, incapable of forming a rational decision.

Endless Debate

There are two main arguments against legalising euthanasia: that severe pain can and should be controlled by drugs; that if doctors are permitted to 'kill' by law, the provision may be abused and people put to death for reasons divorced to mercy. Some of the doctors, especially those who have seen or experienced human suffering concede that there are excruciatingly painful circumstances in which life may be terminated. They feel that a person should have a right to die. However, they also suggest that to minimise the chances of human error and to ensure that no mistake is made and ground cleared for any possibility of abuse or misuse of provisions, acts of omission and or commission leading to mercy killing should be approved by a panel of atleast three specialists, a neurosurgeon or a neurophysician, an ethics committee member or a social worker and a close responsible relation or well wisher of the individual.

Some Experts Caution:

> "in the guise of sanction for mercy killing, monetary temptations are a grave danger. Legislation is no answer. For, there is no such thing as a perfect legislation as there is no such thing as perfect justice. In the ultimate analysis, who shall be the judge? The best of judges can be mistaken."[249]

Infact, with advancement of science, judges find themselves in a dilemma when faced with questions concerning possibility of

[249]Per Justice B Lentin, See, *supra* n 230.

life of a suffering victim. In a Canadian case,[250] the court was concerned with a year old brain damaged child suffering from meningitis where question whether an operation to revise a 'shunt,' a plastic tube which drains excess cerebrospinal fluid away from the brain which had become blocked, should be performed. The parents were opposed to surgery on the reasonging that the boy be allowed to die in dignity rather than live in agony. Evidence showed that without the shunt revision, a boy would not necessarily die but might live for months or years. The Canadian Court however ordered surgery observing that it was too simplistic to say that the child should be allowed to die in peace.

Thus does eternal enigma continue to haunt humankind. Question remains: can there be a justifiable reason for death outside of armed conflict or in self defence? There is no answer yet although mercy killing is spoken of as "morally defendable when it is to put one out of pain by *coup de grace* or glow of mercy."[251]

While this ethico-legal dilemma whether one should attempt to do good to a greatest number or prolong life at all costs in a few rages, the ultimate outcome is gloomy and in any case non-productive. In this tug of war, to permit or not to permit, it is necessary that we balance the need by not being swayed by emotions and at the same time not prolonging life at all costs, because quality of life is as important as the years.

Let no man put assunder,
the handicraft of the Creator,
He is the Giver, He the Receiver,
He the Master Planner,
who shall dare to raise a finger?

---

[250]Re S D (1983) 3 WWR 597, 619. See The Rt Hon Sir John Balcombe, "The Child, the Doctor and the Judge," *Journal of the Royal Society of Medicine* 1996 89/ Suppl 28, 3-9.

[251]M Hidayatullah, *Miscellanea* 156 (1988) N.M.Tripathi Ltd, Mumbai.

Epilogue

The medical scientists and researchers have been working round the clock in their desire to serve humanity and have, time and again, given to world rarest of rare gifts in the form of innovations which have, apart from enhancing life span, improved quality of human life. However, quite a few of these gifts, no sooner given, are turned into curses through filthy materialism and crime that have enveloped society, endangering quality of life of poor masses as also the very lives of the affluent. Although misuse of scientific innovations goes against the very grain of constitutional right to health care which forms part of "obligations cast on government in a welfare state"[252] and the State has displayed its concern for health and safety of its citizens by various legislative and administrative invasions, but the pace has proved to be too tardy and ineffective to meet challenges faced by increased crimes and delayed justice almost to the point of total breakdown.

Advancement of medical science and technology that lent fresh hope to childless couples enabling them to enjoy parenthood and keep their family genes alive through embryo preservation, artificial insemination, test tube babies and the like. However what started off as a laboratory innovation to bring light into human lives, almost immediately misfired into dangerous unethical anti-social game of commercialisation of reproductive organs, poor and needy being easy targets on the chess board.

---

[252]See, *Paschim Banga Khet Mazdoor Samity and others v State of W.B.*, (1996) 4 SCC 37, at 43-44.

While precious lives were sought to be saved through transplant of human organs from dead, a wonderful innovation of science, even before this progressive stride could enter portals of medical history, from the back door entered smugglers and unscrupulous middlemen, creating a worldwide market for human organs, giving rise to kidnappings and fraudulent removals even in hospitals and nursing homes where poor masses entered to gain succour but left *sans* an organ, a loss which they knew nothing about. Unfortunately, a few qualified but mostly fake doctors were also tempted by big monies involved and thus unscrupulous commercial giants could easily make hay with the sun shining bright. Media was the only body which did take half hearted notice but law lords and stickers to the chairs of power could not care less.

Today, on the one hand lie menacing complexities of issues raised as incidental to bio-technological advancement in medical science and on the other, the general mentality of humankind in a fast changing world which has diverted from old established norms of blind faith and worship.

In the Indian scenario, traditions had prevailed, whereby, imparting of information or discussions on disease as well as pros and cons of medical treatment were unknown. The patient accepted what a doctor prescribed. No questions were asked and no commitments made

However change is the law of nature. As in every other sphere, doctors are now encountering more information seeking patients emphasising on clarity and also claiming accountability from a doctor. They are no longer willing to be made scape goats or to be by-passed as innocuous in their own medical procedures. The growing importance of informed consent, even within a doctor - patient equation, not merely for surgical procedures but also conservative treatment, has raised issues co-related to medico-legal ethics, expecting medical fraternity not only to continue maintaining high ethical standards but compelling them to be abreast of legal requirements. One has to appreciate , that this equation has not grown or flourished in a vacuum. It has been enriched by many factors which include time, economics, medical training, current cultural practices in health care and illness management, local peer competition, *et al.* If continuation of a healthy doctor-patient understanding is to be achieved, time is ripe for addressing each of these issues, individually and collectively. A healthy crop cannot be expected out of a blanketed relation based on the magic wand syndrome of blind implicit faith and non-questioning patients. Doctors have to move with times and broadly accept that past standards of keeping patient in blissful ignorance of the disease or imparting partial information to semi-illiterate ones, however laudable the underlying motives, are no longer sustainable. Gone are the days when "Doctor X's red coloured capsules" or "Doctor's blood coloured mixture" were the key-treatment for all ills and diseases, though they may have worked with miraculous healing powers. With progressive society, the scenario has changed. While it is wonderful to be living in this era with man entering nature's arenas and performing miraculous feats, it does bring in added cultures and responsibilities too.

Of course, one cannot over look the other side of the coin. With uncontrolled population explosion renting the nation and ever-depleting proportion of doctors with illegal immigrant masses filling pavements and slums day after day, an over busy doctor can hardly find time to discuss intricacies of each medication with every patient and maintain records of discussions, instructions etc. Economics of time *versus* amount paid to a general practitioner by a single patient make such requirements look ridiculous, what with the ever-rising cost of living and frightening inflation of today. A doctor has naturally to attempt attending to a greater number of patients if he has to end his day with sufficient amount within his pocket to keep his expenses going in accordance with the 'status' which his profession demands.

If one has to take into consideration a pragmatic situation within India where doctors function with greater limitations and in money tight environment as compared to their peer groups in developed countries, it does appear that an unjust step like inflicting accountability within an inappropriate legislation meant for traders dealing with inanimate objects and professing to impart speedy justice in cheap and informal proceedings, with media taking over adjudication of the matter while the case is subjudice, is a situation for which Indian citizenry is not yet geared up. For, in effect, if 'doctor *sahab*' is disgruntled and keeps his cautionary mantles opened up, adverse effects are bound to fall on those in need of relief from their agonising pain and anguish.

In any case, for the medical fraternity, with the air of global accountability creating cyclonic breezes, the change in perception right from days of student training must invade their present existence too. Curriculum of medical colleges now needs to include medico-legal and medico-ethical subjects emphasising record keeping and clarity in documentation etc, as information requirement of a patient now holds as much importance as age-old subjects of anatomy and physiology. Besides, seminars for inculcating communication skills in medical students during college days would equip them with science of 'what' to tell the patient, 'how' to tell the substance, 'how much' to reveal and what 'time' to select for communication, keeping in mind sensitivity of the sick humankind with which doctors are confronted all the time.

Still, the sick, consumer activist and judiciary cannot escape the observations of Sir John Donaldson MR:

"Medicine is not now, and never has been, an exact science. Despite the exercise of the greatest skill, things can go wrong."[253]

---

[253]Supra n 68.

All said and done, the environment today prevalent in our nation is hardly conducive to any one field remaining free from the onslaught, of spreading crime and corruption with morals fully in tact. Still, the medical fraternity has by and large, fulfilled its role well and is still attempting to do its bit towards enriching human lives. It is indeed the lawyer who must now rise to the needs of the nation and its suffering masses and guide the nation to a legal world which bars the pathways to crime, the root cause of today's dilemma. It is the lawyer who, with his vigilance and expertise, must aid the legislature to introduce laws to block the misuse of medical innovations intended to benefit humankind, before they are polluted, and to seal all lucrative routes to acquisition of wealth by criminals, smugglers and unscrupulous. With the politics of the nation having fallen into the hands of many unworthies and illiterates, criminals and corrupt, during the past two decades, it is the lawyer who must come to the nation's rescue by guiding the legal stream in the right direction, attempting to plug the loop holes, as far as possible, in laws imparting justice. It is only by bringing to book the guilty expeditiously, and reducing, if not removing, crime and corruption from the nation through systematised legalistics and a strong executive to enforce implementation that the nation can march ahead towards its goal: Peace and prosperity for all its citizens.

APPENDIX A

Part A - The Indian Contract Act, 1872

S.11 Every person is competent to contract who is of the age of majority according to the law to which he is subject, and who is of sound mind and is not disqualified from contracting by any law to which he is subject.

S.13 Two or more persons are said to consent when they agree upon the same thing in the same sense.

S.14 Consent is said to be free when it is not caused by -

(1) coercion, as defined in section 15, or

(2) undue influence, as defined in section 16, or

(3) fraud, as defined in section 17, or

(4) misrepresentation, as defined in section 18, or

(5) mistake, subject to the provisions of sections 20, 21 and 22.

Consent is said to be so caused when it would not have been given but for the existence of such coercion, undue influence, fraud, misrepresentation or mistake.

S.15 "Coercion" is the committing, or threatening to commit, any act forbidden by the Indian Penal Code (45 of 1860), or the unlawful detaining, or threatening to detain, any property, to the prejudice of any person whatever, with the intention of causing any person to enter into an agreement.

Explanation: It is immaterial whether the Indian Penal Code is or is not in force in the place where the coercion is employed.

S.16 (1) A contract is said to be induced by "undue influence" where the relations subsisting between the parties are such that one of the parties is in a position to dominate the will of the other and uses that position to obtain an unfair advantage over the other.

(2) In particular and without prejudice to the generality of the foregoing principle, a person is deemed to be in a position to dominate the will of another-

(a) where he holds a real or apparent authority over the other, or where he stands in fiduciary relation to the other; or

(b) where he makes a contract with a person whose mental capacity is temporarily or permanently affected by reason of age, illness, or mental or bodily distress.

(3) Where a person who is in a position to dominate the will of another, enters into a contract with him, and the transaction appears, on the face of it or on the evidence adduced, to be inconscionable, the burden of proving that such contract was not induced by undue influence shall lie upon the person in a position to dominate the will of the other.

Nothing in this sub-section shall affect the provisions of section 111 of the Indian Evidence Act, 1872(1 of 1872).

S. 17 "Fraud" means and includes any of the following acts committed by a party to a contract, or with his connivance, or by his agent, with intent to deceive another party thereto or his agent, or to induce him to enter into the contract:-

(1) the suggestion, as a fact, of that which is not true, by one who does not believe it to be true;

(2) the active concealment of a fact by one having knowledge or belief of the fact;

(3) a promise made without any intention of performing it;

(4) any other act fitted to deceive;

(5) any such act or omission as the law specially declares to be fraudulent.

Explanation : Mere silence as to facts likely to affect the willingness of a person to enter into a contract is not fraud, unless the circumstances of the case are such that, regard being had to them, it is the duty of the person keeping silence to speak, or unless his silence is, in itself equivalent to speech.

S. 18 "Misrepresentation" means and includes—

(1) the positive assertion, in a manner not warranted by the information of the person making it, of that which is not true, though he believes it to be true;

(2) any breach of duty which, without an intent to deceive, gains an advantage to the person committing it, or any one claiming under him, by misleading another to his prejudice, or to the prejudice of any one claiming under him;

(3) causing, however innocently a party to an agreement to make a mistake as to the substance of the thing which is the subject of the agreement.

S. 19 When consent to an agreement is caused by coercion, fraud or misrepresentation, the agreement is a contract voidable at the option of the party whose consent was so caused.

A party to a contract, whose consent was caused by fraud or misrepresentation, may, if he thinks fit, insist that the contract shall be performed, and that he shall be put in the position in which he would have been if the representations made had been true.

Exception - If such consent was caused by misrepresentation or by silence, fraudulent within the meaning of section 17, the contract, nevertheless, is not voidable, if the party whose consent was so caused had the means of discovering the truth with ordinary diligence.

Explanation - A fraud or misrepresentation which did not cause the consent to a contract of the party on whom such fraud was practised, or to whom misrepresentation was made, does not render a contract voidable.

Part B - Indian Penal Code, 1860

S. 87 **Act not intended and not known to be likely to cause death or grievous hurt, done by consent.**- Nothing which is not intended to cause death, or grievous hurt, and which is not known by the doer to be likely to cause death or grievous hurt, is an offence by reason of any harm which it may cause, or be intended by the doer to cause, to any person, above eighteen years of age, who has given consent, whether express or implied, to suffer that harm; or by reason of any harm which it may be known by the doer to be likely to cause to any such person who has consented to take the risk of that harm.

S. 88 **Act not intended to cause death, done by consent in good faith for person's benefit.**- Nothing, which is not intended to cause death, is an offence by reason of any harm which it may cause, or be intended by the doer to cause, or be known by the doer to be likely to cause, to any person for whose benefit it is done in good faith, and who has given a consent, whether express or implied, to suffer that harm, or to take the risk of that harm.

S.89 **Act done in good faith for benefit of child or insane person, by or by consent of guardian.**- Nothing which is done in good faith for the benefit of a person under twelve years of age, or of unsound mind, by or by consent, either express or implied, of the guardian or other person having lawful charge of that person, is an offence by reason of any harm which it may cause, or be intended by the doer to cause or be known by the doer to be likely to cause to that person:

Provided -

Provisos.- *First* - That this exception shall not extend to the intentional causing of death, or to the attempting to cause death;

Secondly - That this exception shall not extend to the doing of anything which the person doing it knows to be likely to cause death, for any purpose other than the preventing of death or grievous hurt, or the curing of any grievous disease or infirmity;

Thirdly.- That this exception shall not extend to the voluntary causing of grievous hurt, or to the attempting to cause grievous hurt, unless it be for the purpose of preventing death or grievous hurt, or the curing or any grievous disease or infirmity;

Fourthly - That this exception shall not extend to the abetment of any offence, to the committing of which offence it would not extend.

S.90 **Consent known to be given under fear or misconception.**- A consent is not such a consent as is intended by any section of this Code, if the consent is given by a person under fear of injury, or under a misconception of fact, and if the person doing the act knows, or has reason to believe, that the consent was given in consequence of such fear or misconception; or

Consent of insane person.- if the consent is given by a person who, from unsoundness of mind, or intoxication, is unable to understand the nature and consequence of that to which he gives his consent; or

Consent of child.- unless the contrary appears from the context, if the consent is given by a person who is under twelve years of age.

S.91 **Exclusion of acts which are offences independently of harm caused.**-

The exception in Sections 87, 88 and 89 do not extend to

acts which are offences independently of any harm which they may cause, or be intended to cause, or be known to be likely to cause, to the person giving the consent, or on whose behalf the consent is given.

S.92 **Act done in good faith for benefit of a person without consent.-**

Nothing is an offence by reason of any harm which it may cause to a person for whose benefit it is done in good faith, even without that person's consent, if the circumstances are such that it is impossible for that person to signify consent, or if that person is incapable of giving consent, and has no guardian or other person in lawful charge of him from whom it is possible to obtain consent in time for the thing to be done with benefit:

Provided -

First - That this exception shall not extend to the intentional causing of death, or the attempting to cause death;

Secondly - That this exception shall not extend to the doing of anything which the person doing it knows to be likely to cause death, for any purpose other than the preventing of death or grievous hurt , or the curing of any grievous disease or infirmity;

Thirdly - That this exception shall not extend to the voluntary causing of hurt, or to the attempting to cause hurt, for any purpose other than preventing of death or hurt;

Fourthly - That this exception shall not extend to the abetment of any offence, to the committing of which offence it would not extend.

S.300 Excep 5 Culpable homicide is not murder when the person whose death is caused, being above the age of eighteen years, suffers death or takes the risk of death with his own consent.

S.309 **Attempt to Commit Suicide.-** Whoever attempts to

commit suicide and does any act towards the commission of such offence, shall be punished with simple imprisonment for a term which may extend to one year or with fine, or with both.

Part C - The Consumer Protection Act, 1986

S.2. **Definitions.**-(1) In this Act, unless the context otherwise requires,-

(d) 'consumer' means any person who -

(i)...

(ii) hires or avails of any services for a consideration which has been paid or promised or partly paid and partly promised, or under any system of deferred payment and includes any beneficiary of such services other than the person who hires or avails of the services for consideration paid or promised, or partly paid and partly promised, or under any system of deferred payment, when such services are availed of with the approval of the first mentioned person;

Explanation - For the purpose of sub-clause (i), "commercial purpose" does not include use by a consumer of goods bought and used by him exclusively for the purpose of earning his livelihood, by means of self-employment;

(g) "deficiency" means any fault, imperfection, shortcoming or inadequacy in the quality, nature and manner of performance which is required to be maintained by or under any law for the time being in force or has been undertaken to be performed by a person in pursuance of a contract or otherwise in relation to any service;

(o) "service" means service of any description which is made available to potential users and includes the provision of facilities in connection with banking, financing insurance, transport, processing, supply of electrical or other energy, board or lodging or both, housing construction, entertainment, amusement or the purveying of news of other information, but does not include the rendering of any service free of charge or under a contract of personal service.

Part D - The Transplantation Of Human Organs Act 1994

S.2. In this Act, unless the context otherwise requires,-

(d) "brain-stem death" means the stage at which all functions of the brain-stem have permanently and irreversibly ceased and is so certified under sub-section(6) of section 3;

(f) "donor" means any person, not less than eighteen years of age, who voluntarily authorises the removal of any of his human organs for therapeutic purposes under sub-section (1) or sub-section (2) of section 3;

(h) "human organ" means any part of a human body consisting of a structured arrangement of tissues which, if wholly removed, cannot be replicated by the body;

(i) "near relative" means spouse, son, daughter, father, mother, brother or sister;

(n) "registered medical practitioner" means a medical practitioner who posseses any recognised medical qualification as defined in clause (h) of section 2 of the Indian Medical Council Act, 1956 and who is enrolled on a State Medical Register as defined in clause (k) of that section;

(o) "therapeutic purposes" means systematic treatment of any disease or the measures to improve health according to any particular method or modality; and

(p) "transplantation" means the grafting of any human organ from any living person or deceased person to some other living person for therapeutic purposes.

S.3 Authority for removal of human organs.-

(1) Any donor may, in such manner and subject to such conditions as may be prescribed, authorise the removal, before his death, of any human organ of his body for therapeutic purposes.

(2) If any donor had, in writing and in the presence of two or more witnesses (at least one of whom is a near relative of such person), unequivocally authorised at any time before his death, the removal of any human organ of his body, after his death, for therapeutic purposes, the person lawfully in possession of the dead body of the donor shall, unless he has any reason to believe that the donor had subsequently revoked the authority aforesaid, grant to a registered medical practitioner all reasonable facilities for the removal, for therapeutic purposes, of that human organ from the dead body of the donor.

(3) Where no such authority as is referred to in sub-section (2), was made by any person before his death but no objection was also expressed by such person to any of his human organs being used after this death for therapeutic purposes, the person lawfully in possession of the dead body of such person may, unless he has reason to believe that any near relative of the deceased person has objection to any of the deceased person's human organs being used for therapeutic purposes, authorise the removal of any human organ of the deceased person for its use for therapeutic pruposes.

(4)....

(5) Where any human organ is to be removed from the body of a deceased person, the registered medical practitioner shall satisfy himself, before such removal, by a personal examination of the body from which any human organ is to be removed, that life is extinct in such body or, where it appears to be a case of brain-stem death, that such death has been certified under sub-section (6).

(6) Where any human organ is to be removed from the body

of a person in the event of his brain-steam death, no such removal shall be undertaken unless such death is certified, in such form and in such manner and on satisfaction of such conditions and requirements as may be prescribed, by a Board of medical experts consisting of the following, namely:-

(i) the registered medical practitioner in charge of the hospital in which brain-stem death has occurred;

(ii) an independent registered medical practitioner, being a specialist, to be nominated by the registered medical practitioner specified in clause (i), from the panel of names approved by the Appropriate Authority;

(iii) a neurologist or a neurosurgeon to be nominated by the registered medical practitioner specified in clause (i), from the panel of names approved by the Appropriate Authority; and

(iv) the registered medical practitioner treating the person whose brain-steam death has occurred.

S.4 Removal of human organs not to be authorised in certain cases.-

(1) No facilities shall be granted under sub-section (2) of section 3 and no authority shall be given under sub-section (3) of that section for the removal of any human organ from the body of a deceased person, if the person required to grant such facilities, or empowered to give such authority, has reason to believe that an inquest may be required to be held in relation to such body in pursuance of the provisions of any law for the time being in force.

(2) No authority for the removal of any human organ from the body of a deceased person shall be given by a person to whom such body has been entrusted solely for the purpose of interment, cremation or other disposal.

S.5 Authority for removal of human organs in case of unclaimed bodies in hospital or prison.-

(1) In the case of a dead body lying in a hospital or prison and not claimed by any of the near relatives of the deceased person within forty-eight hours from the time of the death of the concerned person, the authority for the removal of any human organ from the dead body which so remains unclaimed may be given, in the prescribed form, by the person in charge, for the time being, of the management or control of the hospital or prison, or by an employee of such hospital or prison authorised in this behalf by the person in charge of the management or control thereof.

(2) No authority shall be given under sub-section (1) if the person empowered to give such authority has reason to believe that any near relative of the deceased person is likely to claim the dead body even though such near relative has not come forward to claim the body of the deceased person within the time specified in sub-section(1).

S.6 **Authority for removal of human organs from bodies sent for post mortem examination for medicolegal or pathological purposes** - Where the body of a person has been sent for post-mortem examination,-

(a) for medico-legal purposes by reason of the death of such person having been caused by accident or any other unnatural cause; or

(b) for pathological purposes,

the person competent under this Act to give authority for the removal of any human organ from such dead body may, if he has reason to believe that such human organ will not be required for the purpose for which such body has been sent for post-mortem examination, authorise the removal, for therapeutic purposes, of that human organ of the deceased person provided that he is satisfied that the deceased person had not expressed, before his death, any objection to any of his human organs being used, for therapeutic purposes after his death or, where he had granted an authority for the use of any of his human organs for therapeutic purposes after his death, such authority had not been revoked by him before his death..

S.7 **Preservation of human organs.-** After the removal of any human organ from the body of any person, the registered medical practitioner shall take such steps for the preservation of the human organ so removed as may be prescribed.

S. 9. **Restrictions on removal and transplantation of human organs.-**

(1) Save as otherwise provided in sub-section (3), no human organ removed from the body of a donor before his death shall be transplanted into a recipient unless the donor is a near relative of the recipient.

(2).........

(3) If any donor authorises that removal of any of his human organs before his death under sub-section (2) of section 3 for transplantation into the body of such recipient, not being a near relative, as is specified by the donor by reason of affection or attachment towards the recipient or for any other special reasons, such human organ shall not be removed and transplanted without the prior approval of the Authorisation Committee.

(4) (a) The Central Government shall constitute, by notification, one or more Authorisation Committees consisting of such members as may be nominated by the Central Government on such terms and conditions as may be specified in the notification for each of the Union territories for the purposes of this section.

(b) The State Government shall constitute, by notification, one or more Authorisation Committees consisting of such members as may be nominated by the State Government on such terms and conditions as may be specified in the notification for the purposes of this section.

(5) On an application jointly made, in such form and in such manner as may be prescribed, by the donor and the recipient, the Authorisation Committee shall, after holding an inquiry and after satisfying itself that the applicants have complied with all the requirements of this Act and the rules made thereunder, grant to the applicants approval for the removal and transplantation of the human organ.

(6) If, after the inquiry and after giving an opportunity to the applicants of being heard, the Authorisation Committee is satisfied that the applicants have not complied with the requirements of this Act and the rules made thereunder, it shall, for reasons to be recorded in writing, reject the application for approval.

S.14. **Registration of hospitals.-**

(1) No hospital shall commence any activity relating to the removal storage or transplantation of any human organ for therapeutic purposes after the commencement of this Act unless such hospital is duly registered under this Act:

Provided that every hospital engaged, either partly or exclusively, in any activity relating to the removal, storage or tranplantation of any human organ for therapeutic purposes immediately before the commencement of this Act, shall apply for registration within sixty days from the date of such commencement:

Provided further that every hospital engaged in any activity relating to the removal, storage or transplantation of any human organ shall cease to engage in any such activity on the expiry of three months from the date of commencement of this Act unless such hospital has applied for registration and is so registered or till such application is disposed of, whichever is earlier.

S.15 **Certificate of Registration.-**

(1) The Appropriate Authority shall, after holding an inquiry and after satisfying itself that the applicant has complied with all

the requirements of this Act and the rules made thereunder, grant to the hospital a certificate of registration in such form, for such period and subject to such conditions as may be prescribed.

S. 16 **Suspension or cancellation of registration.-**

(1) The Appropriate Authority may, *suo moto* or on complaint, issue a notice to any hospital to show cause why its registration under this Act should not be suspended or cancelled for the reasons mentioned in the notice.

(2) If, after giving a reasonable opportunity of being heard to the hospital, the Appropriate Authority is satisfied that there has been a breach of any of the provisions of this Act or the rules made thereunder, it may, without prejudice to any criminal action that it may take against such hospital, suspend its registration for such period as it may think fit or cancel its registration :

Provided that where that Appropriate Authority is of the opinion that it is necessary or expedient so to do in the public interest, it may, for reasons to be recorded in writing, suspend the registration of any hospital without issuing any notice.

S.18. **Punishment for removal of human organ without authority.-** (1) Any person who renders his services to or at any hospital and who, for purposes of transplantation, conducts, associates with, or helps in any manner in, the removal of any human organ without authority, shall be punishable with imprisonment for a term which may extend to five years and with fine which may extend to ten thousand rupees.

(2) Where any person convicted under sub-section (1) is a registered medical practitioner, his name shall be reported by the Appropriate Authority to the respective State Medical Council for taking necessary action including the removal of his name from the register of the Council for a period of two years for the first offence and permanently for the subsequent offence.

S. 19. **Punishment for commercial dealings in human organs.**- Whoever -

(a) makes or receives any payment for the supply of, or for an offer to supply, any human organ;

(b) seeks to find a person willing to supply for payment any human organ;

(c) offers to supply any human organ for payment;

(d) initiates or negotiates any arrangement involving the making of any payment for the supply of, or for an offer to supply; any human organ;

(e) takes part in the management or control of a body of persons, whether a society, firm or company, whose activities consist of or include the initiation or negotiation of any arrangement referred to in clause (d); or

(f) publishes or distributes or causes to be published or distributed any advertisement,-

(a) inviting persons to supply for payment of any human organ;

(b) offering to supply any human organ for payment; or

(c) indicating that the advertiser is willing to initiate or negotiate any arrangement referred to in clause (d),

shall be punishable with imprisonment for a term which shall not be less than two years but which may extend to seven years and shall be liable to fine which shall not be less than ten thousand rupees but may extend to twenty thousand rupees:

Provided that the court may, for any adequate and special reason to be mentioned in the judgment, impose a sentence of imprisonment for a term of less than two years and a fine less than ten thousand rupees.

Part E - The Transplantation of Human Organs Rules, 1995

R. 4. Duties of the Medical Practitioner.-

(1) A registered medical practitioner shall, before removing a human organ from the body of a donor before his death satisfy himself-

(a) that the donor has given his authorisation in Form 1;

(b) that the donor is in proper state of health and is fit to donate the organ, and shall sign a certificate a specified in Form 2;

(c) that the donor is a near relative of the recipient, and shall sign a certificate as specified in Form 3 after carrying out the following tests on the donor and the recipient, namely :-

(i) tests for the antigenic products of the Human Major Histocompatibility system HLA-A, HLA-B and HLA-DR using conventional serological techniques;

(ii) tests to establish HLA-DR beta and HLADQ beta gene restriction fragment length polymorphism;

(iii) where the tests referred to in sub-clause (i) and sub-clause (ii) do not establish a genetic relationship between the donor and the recipient tests to establish DNA polymorphisms using at least two multi-locus gene probe;

(iv) where the tests referred to in sub-clause (iii) do not establish a genetic relationship between the donor and the recipient further tests to establish DNA polymorphysms using at least five single locus polymorphic probes.

(d) in case recipient is a spouse of the donor, record the statements of the recipient and the donor to the effect that, that are so related and shall sign a certificate in Form 4.

(2) A registered medical practitioner shall, before removing a human organ from the body of a person after his death satisfy

himself-

(a) that the donor had, in the presence of two or more witnesses (at least one of whom is a near relative of such person), unequivocally authorised as specified in Form 5 before his death, the removal of the human organ of his body, after his death, for therapeutic purposes and there is no reason to believe that the donor had subsequently revoked the authority aforesaid;

(b) that the person lawfully in possession of the dead body has signed a certificate as specified in Form 6 or Form 7.

(3) A registered medical practitioner shall, before removing a human organ from the body of a person in the event of his brain-stem death, satisfy himself -

(a) that a certificate as specified in Form 8 has been signed by all the members of the Board of medical experts referred to in sub-section (6) of section 3 of the Act;

(b) that in the case of brain-stem death of a person of less than eighteen years of age, a certificate specified in Form 8 has been signed by all the members of the Board of medical experts referred to in sub-section (6) of section 3 of the Act and an authority as specified in Form 9 has been signed by either of the parents of such person.

R.5. **Preservation of organs.-** The organ removed shall be preserved according to current and accepted scientific methods in order to ensure viability for the purpose of transplantation.

Part F - Motor Vehicles Act, 1988

S.8 **Grant of learner's licence.-**

(3) Every application under sub-section (1) shall be accompanied by a medical certificate in such form as may be prescribed by the Central Government and signed by such registered medical practitioner, as the State Government or any person

authorised in this behalf by the State Government may, be notification in the Official Gazette, appoint for this purpose.

(4) If, from the application or from the medical certificate referred to in sub-section (3), it appears that the applicant is suffering from any disease or disability which is likely to cause the driving by him of a motor vehicle of the class which he would be authorised by the learner's licence applied for to drive to be a source of danger to the public or to the passengers, the licensing authority shall refuse to issue the learner's licence:

Provided that a learner's licence limited to driving an invalid carriage may be issued to the applicant, if the licensing authority is satisfied that he is fit to drive such a carriage.

Appendix B

GLOSSARY

Assault: S.351 of IPC:

Whoever makes any gesture, or any preparation intending or knowing it to be likely that such gesture or preparation will cause any person present to apprehend that he who makes that gesture or preparation is about to use criminal force to that person, is said to commit an assault.

Benefit:

Any act for the good of the patient excluding, however, from its ambit, any pecuniary advantage.

Colles' Fracture:

Fracture of the distal end of radius (long bone of the forearm).

Criminal Force: S.350 of IPC :

Whoever intentionally uses force to any person, without that person's consent, in order to the committing to any offence, or intending by the use of such force to cause, or knowing it to be likely that by the use of such force he will cause injury, fear or annoyance to the person to whom the force is used, is said to use criminal force to that other.

Epilepsy:

Paroxysmal and transitory disturbance of the functions of the brain which develops suddenly, ceases spontaneously and exhibits a conspicuous tendency to recur.

Ejusdem Generis:

The latin phrase "ejusdem generis" means "of the same kind."

Expert Evidence: S.45 Indian Evidence Act, 1872 states:

When the Court has to form an opinion upon a point of foreign law or of science or art, or as to identity of handwriting...the opinions upon that point of persons specially skilled in such foreign law, science or art, or in questions as to identity of handwriting or finger impressions are relevant facts. Such persons are called experts.

Fiduciary Relation:

Includes the relation of a minor and guardian, trustee and the beneficiary, husband and a wife.

Generalised Lymphadenopathy:

Localised or generalised enlargement of the lymph glands accompanied at times, with local heat, tenderness and fever.

Good Faith: S.52 of the IPC states

Nothing is said to be done or believed in "good faith" which is done or believed without due care and attention.

Grievous Hurt: S.320 of the IPC states:

The following kinds of hurt only are designated as "grievous."

First - Emasculation

Secondly - Permanent privation of the sight of either eye.

Thirdly - Permanent privation of the hearing of either ear.

Fourthly - Privation of any member or joint.

Fifthly - Destruction or permanent impairing of the powers of any member or joint.

Sixthly - Permanent disfiguration of the head or face.

Seventhly - Fracture or dislocation of a bone or tooth.

Eightly - Any hurt which endangers life or which causes the sufferer to be during the space of twenty days in severe bodily pain, or unable to follow his ordinary pursuits.

'Harm': The term harm is not well defined in Penal Code; however, S.44 states:

The word 'injury' denotes any harm whatever illegally caused to any person, in body, mind, reputation or property.

Herpes Zoster:

A unilateral inflammatory veiscobullous eruption caused by a virus which attacks the posterior root ganglion and produces the skin eruption secondarily along a cranial or spinal nerve.

Intention:

Purpose or desire to bring about a contemplated result or foresight that certain consequences will follow from the conduct of the person.

Panchnama: First information report.

Pneumonia:

Diseases in which there is an inflammatory consolidation of the lungs.

Pruritic dermatitis:

Characterised by pruritic chronic eruption with inflammatory reaction of the skin.

Voidable:

That which is not *per se* invalid but which can be invalidated or nullified at the option of one of the parties.

Voluntarily Causing Grievous Hurt: S.322 of the IPC states:

whoever voluntarily causes hurt, if the hurt which he intends to cause or knows himself to be likely to cause is grievous hurt, and if the hurt which he causes is grievous hurt, is said "voluntarily to cause grievous hurt".

Explanation: A person is not said voluntarily to cause grievous hurt, except when he both causes grievous hurt and intends or knows himself to be likely to cause grievous hurt. But he is said voluntarily to cause grievous hurt. if, intending or knowing himself to be likely to cause grievous hurt of one kind, he actually causes grievous hurt of another kind.

APPENDIX -C

Opinion Poll Result / at South Mumbai

Letters issued :Consultants : C (200) / General Practitioners : G.P.(200)

Replies received :C (66) / G.P. (51)

	Question		Yes	No
1.	In your opinion, should the doctors have been made liable under the Consumer Protection Act, 1986 (CPA)?	C G.P.	10 14	41 50
2.	Do you think the forums as sanctioned are suitable for imparting justice to doctors?	C G.P.	3 9	46 56
3.	Has the Supreme Courts decision affected the doctor patient equation adversely?	C G.P.	41 55	10 7
4.	In your opinion, has the litigation against doctors been on the increase after clamping of the CPA?	C G.P.	47 58	2 8
5.	According to you, has the Supreme Court decision made any difference in your accountability to the patients?	C G.P.	16 32	23 41

6.	In your opinion, have the referred investigations increased after the decision?	C G.P.	38 55	11 8
7.	Have you procured for yourself an insurance cover?	C G.P.	45 40	6 26
8.	If yes, was it before the CPA has been clamped on the doctors?	C G.P.	29 25	16 13
9.	In your opinion, could the revamped Medical Councils, clothed with suitable powers, serve the victimised patients justly?	C G.P.	43 51	7 12
10.	Have you come across any false or frivolous complaint against any doctor since the opening up of consumer forums?	C G.P.	33 26	17 36

11. In case you feel that CPA, as brought into force, is not suitable to doctors, what in your opinion is the alternate solution to offer easy, quick and cheap redressal to patients for doctors medical negligence?

11. The opinions range from

    1. Strengthening the Medical Council of India
    2. Resorting to present prevalent provisions of civl and crimial laws
    3. Draft fresh legislation for professionals where, in case of medical provisions doctors should be consulted and involved from the stage of drafting

*Sample field survey conducted by Dr Poornima Advani and her team.

APPENDIX -D

Dear Dr Poornima Advani, 13 July 1997

Thank you for your letter. I enclose a brief message as requested for inclusion in your forth coming book.

If you are considering becoming a surrogate mother think long and hard about it as it can be a life changing experience, and that is not always a change for the better. When surrogacy goes wrong many people are hurt. Things to take into consideration; Can you really carry a child for someone else for nine months and not bond with that baby? Will it hurt your own family? Have you completed your own family as pregnancy and birth can be life threatening? You could suffer major regrets and depression! Can you hand over the child after you have just given birth? The couple have to trust you completely, can you trust them too?

If you do feel you are able to help a childless couple and you succeed in your aims, the feeling of well being and achievement should last you throughout your life time. If you experience lack of self confidence or low esteem, doing such a wonderful selfless act might well change all that. It truly can be a positive experience which could overflow into all other aspects of your life. The feel good factor is almost indescribable. You alone have changed two people's barren lives. Made a couple a family. The benefits are great, if all goes well.

Surrogacy is too emotive an issue to take lightly. It is not for the feint hearted either. You will need to be strong, positive and focussed in order to emerge intact both physically and emotionally.

I hope this will suffice. Good luck with your book

Yours sincerely

Kim Cotton

APPENDIX -E

Toolkit - Tips for the Doctors -

A. The Consumer Protection Act, 1986

The medical man has specific defences in case a complaint is filed against him:

- ***locus standi*** In any litigation, the complainant's *locus standi* before a particular Consumer Forum needs to be established, or else the complaint would *ipso facto* fail as not being maintainable. According to *Blacks' Law Dictionary*, *locus standi* means "a right of appearance in a court of justice or before a legislative body, on a given question." Even in a class action complaint instituted by a consumer organisation, credibility of the complainant needs to be established.

- ***volunti non fit injuria*** A Latin maxim, meaning "voluntary assumption of a risk," the risk here being construed as what any reasonable man would expect in the circumstances, is an important tool for the medical man. Bearing in mind the inherent risk involved in each and every medication and medical procedure, allergies and responses being wholly individualistic causing unexpected reactions to a drug even in conservative treatments this provision assumes great significance for the medical fraternity.

  The risks involved in surgical operations and the accompanying anaesthesia, are much larger and well known. It is on this count that the consent form which a patient is asked to sign pre-surgery includes also, by virtue of the risk involved, a consent to unavoidable complications of the surgery. In case of mishap, a well-informed risk of the surgery and patient's consent to it with full knowledge and conscious application of mind, would form a good defence.

- **Limitation** In cases where the claim is delayed beyond the period of limitation, the complaint would be time barred and would therefore not be maintainable. The CPA does not contain any specific provisions with regard to limitation, therefore the limits embodied in the Limitation Act would apply to complaints filed hereunder. In short, claims for which a civil suit is time barred cannot be agitated before a Redressal Forum.[254]

- **Mixed questions of law and fact** The very basic objectives underlying the Act being cheap and speedy imparting of justice, in an informal manner, the Commission avoids dealing with matters requiring elaborate oral and documentary evidence and extensive examination and cross-examination of witnesses or, in short, complicated legal battles stand excluded. All cases involving mixed questions of law and fact requiring voluminous evidence need to be dealt with by the Civil Courts despite the Act.

- **Want of territorial jurisdiction** The machinery of the consumer redressal agencies is created in a three tier hierarchy with the District Consumer Disputes Redressal Forum at the base line, followed by the Consumer Disputes Redressal Commission at the State level and then, the highest body, the National Consumer Disputes Redressal Commission. All the three forums exercise original jurisdiction for entertaining complaints with a division based on the claim amount. Thus, where the value of the goods or services and the compensation, if any claimed,

[254] *Arjunmal Lodha v. Rajasthan Aavasan Mandal,* 1993 (1) CPR 701.

is less than rupees one lakh, the complaint is to be filed with the district forum; in case of a claim exceeding one lakh but within rupees ten lakhs, with the State Commission; beyond which, with the National Commission.

In keeping with the procedural norms, of rendering justice, the dispute can be decided only by that forum having jurisdiction in the matter which is determined by the area where the initial cause of action arose and its pecuniary limits. The defence that a particular forum does not have jurisdiction to handle the case in issue can be a valid defence in the case of district and state levels but would not arise in the apex body. Such a defence cannot be raked up for the first time before the appellate court if the forum of first adjudication has already tried the matter without the issue of jurisdiction being brought up. Nor is it in the hands of the parties to mutually come to an understanding that a particular forum which does not have the requisite jurisdiction, should handle the case in issue. Likewise, a mutual contract cannot take away an existing jurisdiction of a particular forum.

- ***Res judicata*** The principle of *res judicata* is based on the policy of preventing multiplicity of litigation and agitating the same matter, between the parties, which has already been decided earlier, that is, if a matter is already decided by a civil court, no proceedings will lie under the Consumer Protection Act, 1986 in respect of the same subject matter.[255]

  Although, strictly speaking, the Consumer Redressal Forums are not courts, yet the principle of *res judicata* does govern them on the principle that the CPA simply provides additional forums to the aggrieved parties which they are at liberty to select. But under no circumstance would a matter between the same parties

---

[255] *M/s. Dullar Enterprises Pvt. Ltd v. Punjab National Bank*, 1993 (2) CPR 652 (SCDRC Rajasthan).

decided by a competent civil court, be re-opened and re-adjudicated by the consumer forum. The principles of *res judicata* would operate as a bar.

- **Suppression of material facts** If the complainant suppresses material facts from the Consumer Forums, he would not be entitled to any relief.

In any case, the CPA is not an avenue for every grievance against the doctor. Nor can it be used to ventilate grievances against accidental or incidental mishaps. For example, where a patient suffering from a cat bite approached a hospital for first aid and an anti rabies vaccine was administered but the patient died due to complications arising out of it, it was held to be an 'unfortunate incident for which none could be blamed or held responsible'.[256]

B. Medical Negligence

A discreet medical man would be particularly careful in taking all reasonable precautions against any act or omission which could amount to medical negligence. Some of the very logical precautions would be:

- accurate records to be maintained at every stage;
- clinical examination to be carefully conducted and recorded;
- diagnosis, where required to be confirmed by laboratory tests including biopsy, should not be acted upon till after the investigations;
- x-rays, in case of injury to bones and joints or where diagnosis on clinical examination is doubtful, are a must;
- consultation with a specialist should be recommended only where a specialist in the field can further benefit a patient;

---

[256]*Smt. Dipti De Sarkar v. Steel Authority of India Lt., Rourkela Steel Plant and Ors,* 1993 (1) CPR 640.

- immunisation should be considered where there is a danger of infection;
- sensitivity tests should invariably be conducted before injecting prescribed doses of drugs likely to cause an anaphylactic shock;
- drugs to be administered by injection or otherwise need to be checked;
- no surgery or experimental therapy should be adopted without prior consent;
- no procedures, not in consonance with the qualifications and professional skill, should be undertaken;
- reports should be written or typed as soon as possible. They should indicate the date and the time when they were dictated, or written, and if typed, they should be checked by the physician before signing the same. In legal parlance, a rubber stamp of signature is no proof that the concerned physician has read its contents and would not serve to mitigate the accusations of negligence;
- prognosis should be projected with caution and conservatively;
- attend to all the patients personally; sign all the reports personally, no proxy allowed;
- in case of surgery, perform all the surgical procedures personally without resorting to 'ghost surgery' or, in short, the assistant doing the work with the chief otherwise busy, may be even absent from the operation theatre. A privity of contract has been entered into by the operating surgeon with the patient and he is expected to abide by the terms whatever be his exigencies. However, the anaesthesist, though not engaged directly by the patient but by the surgeon, and is paid the professional fees from the total amount paid by the patient he is independently liable for any adverse effects caused due to

inadvertence in administering anaesthesia;[257]

- do not thrust excessive responsibility on a nurse whether she is capable or not. Under the law of vicarious responsibility, it is the doctor who would be held responsible for any mishap caused by negligence of the nurse;
- check that the entire set of equipments required are handy, properly sterlised where required and in order, before resorting to any surgical procedure;
- ensure that the generator is functioning and is ready to be pressed into service in case of electricity failure in between the operation as such defect in hospital / nursing home services can cause havoc to the patient and is bound to be adjudged as gross negligence. On whom the resultant axe will fall and the quantum of compensation payable will depend on the depositions made before the court and the damage caused to the victim;
- utmost caution in labelling of bottles and solutions is essential. In a case where the patient's left eye was damaged as the doctor put drops of acid instead of eye wash, the doctor was held to be negligent and a compensation of Rs 1,00,000/- was awarded;[258]
- the doctor should refrain from conducting consultations or committing to diagnosis without seeing the patient or suggesting treatment in *absentia*. In case the patient is known to him or is his regular patient, such emergency advice should be backed by regular follow-up;
- in case of a serious patient, the doctor is entitled to a house visit before advising hospitalisation or directing the patient to hospital where he would give a check up;

---

[257]*Mumbai Grahak Panchayat v Dr (Mrs) Rashmi Fadnavis,* 1996 (1) CPR 137.
[258]*K Kuttappan v Beniger Hospital and others,* 1996 (1) CPR 462 (SCDRC, Kerala).

- there are no restrictions to fees charged by a private medical practitioner as the same have been left to the individual's own parameters. In practice, it is in fact impossible to predict as to how much labour and time would be required by an individual patient for any course of treatment as human physiology does not respond equally even in similar circumstances.

C. Planned Babies And Hired Mothers

Doctors handling artificial insemination must make it a point to:

- maintain their records and papers with clarity and utmost secrecy;
- compulsorily obtain a written consent of the husband and the wife for having a baby borne by the surrogate (failure to do so can land the doctor in an accusation of aiding or abetting either of them);
- obtain consent of the husband of the surrogate (of course presuming the consent of the surrogate herself), as it would keep the path clear in case of future accusations and discord between the involved parties;
- devote some time to explaining to the prospective parents and the surrogate, the consequences of the procedure and the state laws on the subject, prior to obtaining the consent of the parties. The fact of the doctor having explained these essentials to the concerned parties must be clearly reflected in the consent form;
- maintain the identity of the donor in the medical records (marked strictly confidential) to prevent complications and to ensure the welfare of the child.
- maintain as confidential the identity of the recipient and the outcome of the venture , in case the donor is other than the prospective father.

- screen for Rh status, HIV infection, thalessemia and any other transmittable disease, the donor as well as the surrogate, to ensure that persons with such diseases are not inducted in the process so that the surrogate and the proposed progeny are safe;
- restrict surrogacy, ethically as well as legally, to married women including widows;
- record the blood group of the donor and surrogate and inform the prospective parents;
- keep all the records handy as he may be required to produce them in a court of law in case of future disputes or contingencies;
- hand over, despite utmost secrecy of identity of the donor, the medical and genetic data of the donor and the surrogate to the prospective parents;

Need for urgent legislation

Following legislatory safeguards are suggested:

- only childless couples where either of the spouse's incapacity to reproduce/ bear a child has been conclusively established should be permitted A.I.D;
- the consent of the husband, the wife and / or the surrogate's husband need to be made mandatory as they are of paramount importance to negate charges of adultery;
- in case of intervention of donor and / or surrogate, legal adoption by the prospective parents must be made compulsory to give the child the stamp of legitimacy and a right to inheritance;
- a special panel of licensed doctors of repute should alone be authorised to deal with cases of genetic engineering.
- legislation for maintenance of record pertaining to surrogacy is essential.

D. AIDS

Health care programmes should include:

- continuing health education and camps especially in the high risk areas.

These camps should aim at:

- providing basic information about the virus and its mode of transmission;
- making the people aware of the deadly consequences of the disease;
- creating awareness about protective methods;
- empowering people to take adequate protective measures themselves.

In addition:

- safe and effective contraceptive care should be provided for all seropositive women because of the known adverse consequences of HIV during pregnancy;
- importance of use of disposable or sterilised syringes by the patient must be highlighted and made compulsory as HIV is destroyed at 65 degrees;
- strict scrutiny in screening of blood before transfusion should be made mandatory;
- WHO recommendation that all asymptomatic HIV infected children should receive standard vaccines, must be implemented;[259]
- when the AIDS patient is to have surgery, the attending surgeon should inform the operating room and also notify the pathology

[259]Ch Suvarna Raju & Mrs Ch Rama Kumari Sahu, "HIV/AIDS and Law Relating To Women and Children" 420, at 433, vol 2, Supra n 184.

laboratory when the specimen is sent there. The label 'caution AIDS' should be placed on the specimen container and wrapped; disposable gowns, sheets etc should be treated as is done for contaminated cases;

- 'positive peoples meetings' should be organised where victims can share their experiences and boost the morale of other sufferers;
- quacks who exploit the ignorance of the public by offering 'magical' remedies for the AIDS patient must be eliminated by harsh measures. Newspapers and other media should caution the masses against such hazards.

To sum up, HIV related laws have to aim at addressing the problems and issues in general and create an environment for facing the challenge posed by the pandemic and more specifically by:

- aiding and channelling resources for surveillance, policy determination and its intervention;
- aiming at education, counselling, treatment and disease management in the interest of general public health and prevention of spread of the disease;
- establishing norms for treating the victims of AIDS, as their basic human right, while specifying their sanctions against them in the interests of general public;
- ensuring compulsory quality control of products such as blood, semen, organs, tissues etc for human consumption and the regularised use of HIV test kits and condoms so that the affected individuals can co-exist with others to ensure a reasonable quality of life.

In any case, prevention of HIV transmission and the minimisation of personal and social impact of HIV should be the basic objectives of HIV/AIDS programmes. This can be attempted through media and framed informative pamphlets which can reach out to the masses educating them at an early stage in life on how to save themselves from the dreaded disease. Laws must play their role well in regulating information broadcast and educational agendas.

Donations of blood, semen or organs are other areas with high risk of spread of infection and therefore areas in which criminal sanctions ought to be provided. It is obviously safer and more cost effective to exclude contaminated blood samples at the outset, yet some countries, including India, where blood donations have been a source of earning for the poor, the blood banks have hardly introduced any cautionary measures so essential to safeguard humanity.

REFERENCES

Cases

A.S. Mittal and anr v State of U.P. and others, (1989) 3 SCC 223.

Achutrao Haribhau Khodwa and others v State of Maharashtra, (1996) 2 SCC 634.

Arjunmal Lodha v Rajasthan Aavasan Mandal, 1993 (1) CPR 701.

B.S. Hegde v Dr Sudhansu Bhattacharya, 1993 (3) CPR 414 (NCDRC).

Bolam v Friern Barnet HMC, (1957)2 All E R 118.

Chatterton v Gerson and another, (1981)1 Ali ER 257.

Common Cause v Union of India and others with Consumer Education and Research Society v Union of India, AIR 1993 SC 1403.

Dharmendra Kumar Mishra v Dr Akhauri S Sinha, 1996 (2) CPR 192.

Smt Dipti De Sarkar v Steel Authority of India Ltd, Rourkela Steel Plant and others, 1993 (1) CPR 640.

M/s Dullar Enterprises Pvt Ltd v Punjab National Bank, 1993 (2) CPR 652 (SCDRC, Rajasthan).

Emeh v Kensington and Chelsea and Westminster Area Health Authority, (1984)3 All ER 1044.

Eyre v Measday, (1986) 1 All ER 488.

Francis Coralie v Delhi Administration, AIR 1981 SC 746.

Gian Kaur v State of Punjab and others, 1996 Cri.LJ 1660 (SC).

Greaves & Co (Contractors) Ltd v Baynham Meikle & Partners, (1975)3 All ER 99.

Hills v Potter and others, (1983)3 All ER 716.

Indian Medical Association v V P Shantha and others, AIR 1996 SC 550.

K. Kuttappan v Beniger Hospital and others, 1996 (1) CPR 462 (SCDRC, Kerala).

K. Raji Reddy v Dr (Mrs) Aruna Reddy, 1996 (1) CPR 244 (SCDRC, A P, Hyderabad).

Kuldip Singh Dhillon v Post Graduate Institute of Medical Education and Research, 1996 (3) CPR 18 (CDRC, UT, Chandigarh).

Dr. Laxman Balkrishna Joshi v Dr. Trimbak Bapu Godbole, AIR 1969 SC 128.

Dr Sr Louie and Anr v Smt Kannolil Pathumma and anr, 1993 (1) CPR 422.

M.L.Singhal v. Dr. Pradeeparthur and anr, AIR 1996 Delhi 261.

Sau Madhuri v Dr Rajendra, (1996) III CPJ 75, 76 (NC).

Maynard v West Midlands Regional Health Authority, (1985) 1 All ER 635.

Mumbai Grahak Panchayat v Dr (Mrs) Rashmi Fadnavis, 1996 (1) CPR 137.

Murray v McMurchy, (1949) 1 All ER 497.

Dr N T Subrahmanyam and anr v Dr B Krishna Rao and anr, 1996 (2) CPR 247 (N.C).

Oxford v Oxford, (1921) 49 Ontario Law Report 22.

P. Rathinam Nagbhusan Patnaik v Union of India, AIR 1994 SC 1844.

Pt Parmanand Katara v Union of India, AIR 1989 SC 2039.

Paschim Banga Khet Mazdoor Samity and others v State of W.B., (1996) 4 SCC 37.

Poonam Verma v Ashwin Patel and others, AIR 1996 SC 2111.

REL v EL, 1949 Probate Division 211.

Ramanand B Raikar v Salgaonkar Medical Research Centre and anr, 1993 (3) CPR 300.

Roe v Minister of Health, (1954)2 QB 66, at 87.

Re S, (1992) 4 All ER 671.

S S Kahlon and Anr v Bawa Hospital, 1994 (1) CPR 773 (SCDRC, Punjab).

Schloendorff v Society of New York Hospital, (1914) 211 NY 125, N.Y.Ct of Apps.

Sidaway v Bethlam Royal Hospital Governors and others, (1984) 1 All ER 1018.

Sunita Vasant Heganawar v Miraj Medical Centre, II (1994)CPJ 544.

Re T, (1992) 4 All ER 649.

Dr T.T. Thomas v Smt Elisa and others, AIR 1987 Kerala 52-56.

Thake v Maurice, (1986) 1 All E.R. 497.

Tukaram v State of Maharashtra, AIR 1979 SC 185.

Articles

Cheryl G. Healton, M Lyndon Haviland and Ram Kairam, "Challenges of AIDS Prevention for Women in Both the Developing and Developed World" vol.2, Proceedings of Interdisciplinary International Conference on AIDS-Law and Humanity, The Indian Law Institute, New Delhi (1995).

Dr.D. Sengupta, "AIDS-Diagnosis and Control", *Swasth Hind* (Nov.-Dec 1990).

G.V. Krishnan, "Batista operation helps the failing heart a better pump", *The Times of India* (Bombay ed) (26 November 1996).

George P. Smith, "Sexual Autonomy or Government Intervention: Artificial Fathers and Surrogate Mothers," World Congress on Law and Medicine, Indian Law Institute (New Delhi, 1985).

The Rt Hon Sir John Balcombe, "The Child, the Doctor and the Judge," *Journal of the Royal Society of Medicine* 1996 89/Suppl 28, 3-9.

L.M. Singhvi, "Need to Redefine Concept of Death," *Times of India* (Bombay ed) 24 February 1992.

M.S. Venkataraman "Kidney Donation-Sacrifice or Trade?" *Legal Aspects of Health Care* (1995) (Indian Society of Health Administrators).

Paras Diwan, "Technological *Niyoga* and *Nirodh* and Social Engineering Through Law" 22 *J.I.L.I.* 445, 449-50 (1980).

Poornima Advani, "Euthanasia: The Eternal Enigma", *The Afternoon Despatch & Courier,* 30 April 1993.

Poornima Advani, "Duty to Care: From Hippocrates to Consumer Forums," paper presented at International Conference on Global Health Laws, New Delhi, 6-7 December 1997.

Richard Lillich, "Legal Regulation of the Sale and Transplantation of Human Organs," paper presented at the World Congress on Law and Medicine, Indian Law Institute, New Delhi, 1985.

Prof. S.R. Bhansali, "Need for Law to Control HIV/AIDS in India" vol.2, Proceedings of Interdisciplinary International Conference on AIDS-Law and Humanity, The Indian Law Institute, New Delhi, 1995.

Tobi Saidel, Bill Rau "Uses of HIV/AIDS Epidemologic Data, Estimates and Projections in Policy Development", vol III, Paper presented at Interdisciplinary International Conference of AIDS - Law and Humanity, Indian Law Institute, New Delhi.

Texts

Barbara Eck Menning, A Guide for the Childless Couple (1977) Prentice Hall Press.

Bernard Knight, Legal Aspects of Medical Practice (1992) Churchill Livingstone.

Bury B, Cook S.A, Adcock F.E.(ed), The Cambridge Ancient History, vol v(Athens 478-401) (1935) Cambridge University Press.

C.A. Franklin (ed), Textbook of Medical Jurisprudence and Toxicology (1988) N.M.Tripathi Publication, Mumbai.

Chamber's 21st Century Dictionary (1997) Allied Chamber's (India) Limited, New Delhi.

Cook S.A., F.E.Adcock, Charlesworth M P (ed), The Cambridge Ancient History, vol ix (The Roman Republic 133-44 B C) (1935) Cambridge University Press.

D.C. Jayasuriya (ed) HIV, Law and Humans Rights - Text and Materials (1995) UNDP Regional Project on HIV and Development.

D.N. Saraf, Law of Consumer Protection in India, 2nd ed.(1995) N.M. Tripathi Pvt. Ltd., Mumbai.

George W. Field, Field's Medico-Legal Guide and Medical Jurisprudence (1988) The University Book Agency, Allahabad.

Harry Keen, John Jarrett, Arthur Levy, Triumphs of Medicine (1976) Paul Elek, Ltd.

Herbert Broom, A Selection of Legal Maxims, 10th ed(1995) Sweet & Maxwell, London.

Homi S.Mehta, Medical Law and Ethics in India (1963) The Bombay Samachar Pvt.Ltd.

J.A. Jolowicz and T.Elliis Lewis (ed), Winfield On Tort 8th ed(1967) Sweet & Maxwell, London.

Joseph Bellina and Josleen Wilson, The Fertility Handbook: A Positive and Practical Guide (1986) Penguin Books.

Keye, Chang, Rebar and Sailes, Infertility Evaluation and Treatment (1995) W B Saunders & Co.

Kim Cotton, Second Time Around (1992) Kim Cotton, New Barnet, Herts.

Lenard R Berlanstein, The Barristers of Toulouse in the Eighteenth Century (1740-1793) (1975) The John Hopkins University Press.

M. Hidayatullah, Miscellanea (1988) N M Tripathi Pvt Ltd., Mumbai.

P.S. Pasricha, You Only Live Once (1995) Nasha Publication, Mumbai.

P V Kane, History of Dharmasastra (Ancient and Medieval Religious and Civil Laws in India) vol 1 (1968) Bhandarkar Oriental Research Institute, Poona.

Panos Dossier, Triple Jeopardy: Women and AIDS (1990) Panos Publication Ltd.

Parikh, Textbook of Medical Jurisprudence and Toxicology, 5th ed(1990) CBS Publishers & Distributors.

Poornima Advani, Causes of Antisocial Behaviour and Crime: A Socio and Medicolegal Perspective, (1990) Gopushi Publishers, Mumbai.

Poornima Advani, Crime in Marriages: A Broad Spectrum (1995) Gopushi Publishers, Mumbai.

R.G. Edwards and Jean M Purdy (ed), Human Conception *In Vitro* (1982) Academic Press Inc.

Ratanlal and Dhirajlal, Law of Crimes, vol.2 (1988) Bharat Law House.

Regina Graycar & Jenny Morgan, The Hidden Gender of Law (1990) The Federation Press.

Robert Duthie, George Bentley (ed)., Mercer's Orthopeadic Surgery 8th ed, (1983) University Park Press, Baltimore.

Robert Franklin and Dorothy Brockman, In Pursuit of Fertility (1991) Henry Holt and Co., New York.

Robert Glick, Law, Ethics and HIV (1993) UNDP Regional Project.

Roderick E. McGrow, Encyclopaedia of Medical History (1985) Macmillan Press, London.

Ruth Montgomery, A World Beyond (Fawcett Publication, Inc. Greenwich, Conn.)

Sanjiva Rao, The Advocates Act and the Legal Practitioners Act (1987) The Law Book Company (Pvt) Ltd, Allahabad.

Smith William, Christian Antiquities vol.1 (1875) John Murray, London.

(Dr) Tony Smith(ed), The British Medical Association: Complete Family Health Encyclopaedia (1996) Dorling Kinderley.

The Holy Bible.

Newspapers

Business Standard (Calcutta ed) 16 April 1995.

Haj News, 1 April 1995.

Savvy (Bombay ed) October 1995.

Sunday Observer, 5 November 1995.

Sunday Observer, 18 August 1996.

The Afternoon Despatch & Courier (Bombay ed) 1 December 1997.

The Daily (Bombay ed) 8 November 1995.

The Daily (Bombay ed) 7 December 1996.

The Hindu (Madras ed) 26 November 1996.

The Hindu (New Delhi) 12 August 1997.

The Hindu (New Delhi) 21 October 1997.

The Hindustan Times (New Delhi) 6 January 1985.

The Independent (Bombay ed) 13 February 1993.

The Pioneer (Delhi ed) 24 February 1994.

The Pioneer (Delhi ed) 5 August 1994.

The Pioneer (Delhi ed) 19 April 1995.

The Pioneer (Delhi ed) 5 October 1996.

The Saturday Statesman (Delhi ed) 15 April 1995.

The Statesman (Delhi ed) 30 November 1996.

The Times of India (Bombay ed) 21 August 1995.

The Times of India (Bombay ed) 15 December 1995.

The Times of India (Bombay ed) 15 November 1996.

The Times of India (New Delhi ed) 22 August 1997.

The Times of India (New Delhi ed) 10 November 1997.

The Times of India (Bombay ed) 2 December 1997.